Through the Gateway of the Heart

Second Edition

Through the Gateway of the Heart

Second Edition

Accounts of Experiences with MDMA and Other Empathogenic Substances

Compiled and Edited by
Sophia Adamson
(*Nom de Plume* of Ralph Metzner & Padma Catell)

Foreword by Ralph Metzner

Preface by Padma Catell

Solarium Press

An Imprint of Castalia Communications
Petaluma, California

Printed in the United States of America.

Library of Congress Control Number: 2012945065

ISBN Number 978-0-929150-79-6

Cover art: "Gift of Light" by Susan Seddon Boulet
Used with permission of the copyright holder.

Published by:
Solarium Press, P.O. Box 2503 Petaluma, CA 94953
An Imprint of Castalia Communications.

Through the Gateway of the Heart

Table of Contents

Preface to the Second Edition

By Padma Catell, Ph.D.

It has been over twenty-seven years since the original edition of this book was published. Regretfully, there has been very little research on using these substances as tools to facilitate psychotherapy since then; although over the years there have been various studies (National Institute on Drug Abuse, 2006; Beitia, Cobreros, Sainz & Cenarruzabeitia, 2000; Ricaurte, Martello, Katz & Martello. 1992; Steele, McCann & Ricaurte, 1994) on the pharmacology and toxicology of 3,4-methylenedioxymethamphetamine (MDMA). It is important to note that the majority of these studies have not been done in humans. It has only been within the last few years, beginning in 2004, that researchers have been able to get permission to explore the therapeutic value of these compounds in legally sanctioned studies.

Before 1985 it was not illegal to use MDMA, which at that time was called "Adam," as an adjunct to psychotherapy. At that time MDMA was not a scheduled drug since it was before the 1985 "designer drug" laws were passed. It is important to note that the substances sold on the street today as "ecstasy" are often not pure and are frequently adulterated with all sorts of other chemicals, some of which are known to be harmful. For complete information and details on adulterants commonly contained in ecstasy tablets and capsules see: http://www.ecstasydata.org/.

Rick Doblin and others at the Multidisciplinary Association for Psychedelic Studies (MAPS) have spent many years working to have studies approved using these compounds. I am happy to state that this approved research is now moving into its next stage, studies with larger numbers of subjects. Currently (2012) there are studies using MDMA going on in the US, Great Britain, Switzerland, and Israel. (For extensive, detailed information and updates on this research, see the MAPS website, www.MAPS.org.)

A Brief History

The first synthesis of MDMA was by Köllisch in 1912 at a German pharmaceutical company, Merck and Company. At that time no specific use was indicated for MDMA (Parker et, al. 1998). There is a more than 25 year-long history of using these types of drugs to facilitate psychotherapy. One early researcher was Dr. George Greer. Dr. Greer did a study with 29 subjects; these people were not his psychotherapy clients (Greer & Tolbert, 1986). He concluded that all of his subjects benefited in a variety of ways. His subjects who had psychological diagnoses reported significant relief from their problems. Dr. Greer believes that because MDMA is not dissociative, subjects can remember and integrate what they have learned during the MDMA state into their everyday behavior. Like most therapists who have done this work, he believes continued psychotherapy is required for the changes to be useful in one's daily life (in Seymour, 1986).

The brief vignettes in this book illustrate the usefulness of these drugs to facilitate insight and healing. I would have liked to visit with the subjects who shared their experiences in the original volume and get an update as to the value of this work looking back with the perspective of twenty-seven years. However, for reasons of confidentiality records of their names were not kept. Judging by reports from a few with whom we are still in contact, their memories of these sessions are intense and poignant even though almost three decades have passed. Many of them report that these experiences remain as some of the most significant events, if not the most significant, in the course of their lives.

Over the last few years, I have come to think that this book was originally published at exactly the wrong time; it came out just when the use of "designer drugs" became illegal (1985) for any purpose, including that of facilitating psychotherapy. Therapists who had been using them in psychotherapy stopped doing so, or went "underground." At this time, when there is a resurgence of interest in their therapeutic use and ongoing legally sanctioned research, it seemed that a second edition of this volume would be appropriate and useful. For more specific information on how to become a psychedelic researcher see http://www.maps.org/resources/students/.

A Note on Terminology

There is an ongoing, friendly debate as to the best term to use in describing MDMA and similar compounds. We prefer the use of the word "empathogen," meaning to generate empathy, as this is the quality that is unique to this group of drugs and the reason they are useful as tools in training potential psychotherapists. Inherent in the experience of empathy is a decrease in "self-centeredness," a state that a psychotherapist must cultivate in order to understand the world from the client's point of view. This understanding is necessary for psychotherapy to be effective.

How Does MDMA Facilitate Psychotherapy?

Over the years it has become clear to me (and many others) that MDMA is a substance that reduces fear. In psychotherapy there is the concept of "resistance." Resistance is usually thought of as the conflict between the motivation within the client that wants to change and the fears that get in the way and prevent the changes. You could also think of these fears as giving rise to many of the defense mechanisms. These defense mechanisms serve to decrease anxiety when a client comes up against material that invokes fear. The usual reason for therapy is to change something that one feels is not useful or is harmful in one's life, but that one has not been able to change on one's own. The blocks to this desired change are the defense mechanisms and/or resistance to therapy in particular.

Somehow MDMA has the unique and almost "magical" power of reducing fear. There is empirical research to show that MDMA reduces activity in the part of the brain called the amygdala (Passie, 2010). This is the part of the brain believed to be at the center of most of the brain events associated with fear. It is also known that MDMA causes a release of serotonin and dopamine in the brain; this effect on the neurotransmitters may also be a part of why fear is lessened (Crespi, Mennini & Gobbi, 1997). When the fear is lessened the client is able to talk about material that is usually defended against in the so-called "normal" state of mind. The action of MDMA allows the client and the therapist access to the material that was defended against, and allows the client to "work through" that material. In other words, the client is able to bring into consciousness material that is usually kept at an unconscious level. Material that is unconscious is not easily amenable to change. If we don't even know what it is, how can we attempt to change it? Change is only possible after the material becomes conscious. It is like trying to solve a problem before one knows/understands what the problem is. This is impossible to do. Once the problem is brought into consciousness, the client can work on a solution.

In this way MDMA (and other similar empathogens) reduce defenses and allows unconscious material to be revealed to the conscious mind and then worked on. This is a process that takes place (one hopes) in the normal course of psychotherapy. The difference is that it can take years before a client feels safe enough to let down unconscious barriers and reveal whatever is causing the problems. This process is both very expensive and very time consuming. As a psychotherapist I would say that it is possible for a typical client to progress as much in one MDMA session as in six months of once-a-week psychotherapy.

The vignettes contained in this volume illustrate a wide variety of experiences, some using MDMA alone, and a few using MDMA with 4-bromo-2,5-dimethoxyphenethylamine (2-CB) an empathogen with similar effects. All of the experiences were aimed at gaining insight. It was the goal of many of the subjects and the guides and therapists working with them that the insights gained during the sessions, with the help of these substances, be retrieved and used in future therapy. The new insights could then be applied to facilitate a change in behavior, or to a greater understanding of oneself. It was hoped that the lessons learned not be lost or forgotten when the subjects returned to their "ordinary" state of mind. For this reason, some of the sessions were recorded, or at times notes were taken by the guide or by the subject, for reference and use in the future.

Guidelines for This Type of Work

The section entitled: *Guidelines for the Sacramental Use of Empathogenic Substances,* (155-171) is a brief description of what we think is important in setting up and running a guided therapeutic session using empathogens. For a detailed treatise on guidelines for this research we refer you to an article published in 2008 in the *Journal of Psychopharmacology*, titled "Human hallucinogen research: Guidelines for safety," (Johnson, Richards & Griffiths, 2008). These guidelines propose recommendations for the safe administration of psychedelic drugs and the minimization of adverse reactions. They were designed for the use of these compounds within a research setting. These guidelines (Johnson, et al.) provide extensive, detailed information about set and setting, the preparation of subjects, and the selection and preparation of support personnel. The authors also review previous research on human subjects and emphasize the value of extensive preparation to decrease the possibility of adverse reactions such as panic or paranoid states and to increase the number of positively valued experiences.

Latest News on Neurotoxicity

Questions about the neurotoxic effects of ecstasy on the brain remain highly topical in light of its popularity among young people. Most of the fear that MDMA/ecstasy could be neurotoxic was generated by a study published in the journal *Science* in 2002 (Ricaurte, et al.). This study was later retracted (2003) when it was discovered that the vials thought to contain MDMA actually contained methamphetamine. No one questions that methamphetamine is neurotoxic. The original study (Ricaurte, et al., 2002) generated lots of publicity while the retraction was hardly noted by the press.

Since then there continue to be studies to evaluate whether MDMA is neurotoxic and what kind, if any, negative long-term effects may occur. The research in humans is very limited, and the number of subjects in the studies is very small.

Much of the recent research on these compounds (empathogens) in the US has focused on the treatment of Post-traumatic Stress Disorder (PTSD). The PTSD Foundation reported in 2007 that one in three returning troops has serious post-traumatic stress symptoms. The Department of Veterans' Affairs estimates that 830,000 Vietnam War veterans suffered PTSD symptoms (not the full DSM IV-TR diagnosis) (in Mintz, 2007). Even now, almost forty years later, four out of five are still reporting symptoms (Mintz, 2007). For many of those, the PTSD symptoms will be a life-long problem. The treatments we currently are using for this disorder are not very effective. They may relieve the symptoms temporarily, but do not treat the underlying disorder, and many people with PTSD do not even respond to the available treatments. Clearly, the need for more effective treatments for PTSD is great.

An example of a study using MDMA for the treatment of chronic PTSD also looked at whether there were any adverse neurocognitive effects or serious adverse drug-related effects (Mithoefer, et al., 2011). This study is the first completed clinical trial evaluating MDMA as a therapeutic adjunct. The twenty patients in the study were diagnosed with chronic post-traumatic stress disorder. These subjects were refractory to both psychotherapy and psychopharmacological interventions. The test subjects received MDMA-assisted psychotherapy. Researchers found the change in PTSD Scale scores from baseline was significantly greater for the group that received MDMA than for the placebo group. The rate of clinical response was 10/12 (83%) in the active treatment group versus 2/8 (25%) in the placebo group. These researchers found no serious drug-related adverse events, no adverse neurocognitive effects, and no clinically significant blood pressure increases. They concluded that there was no evidence that MDMA caused harm to their subjects and that it may be useful in patients refractory to other treatments. These are exciting recent findings using MDMA for the treatment of PTSD, especially in combat veterans (Mithoefer, et al., 2011).

For an extensive review of the literature on neurotoxicity research in humans see the overview by Baggott and Jerome (p.101-145) on the MAPS website. Larger, longitudinal, and prospective studies are still needed in order to obtain a clearer understanding of any possible long-term consequences of MDMA use in humans.

It is hoped that reading the examples of the sessions in this volume will be of value to anyone who wishes to learn about the use and potential of these substances. I believe that reading first-hand, specific instances where people have benefited from the use of empathogens will provide some framework for how they can be used productively in psychotherapy.

References for the Preface

Baggott, M., B.A. & Jerome, L., Ph.D. (2010). Neurotoxicity Research in Humans. http://www.maps.org/research/mdma/protocol/review5.pdf. p101-145.

Beitia, G., Cobreros, A., Sainz, L. & Cenarruzabeitia E. (2000). Ecstasy-induced toxicity in rat liver. *Liver*. 20(1):8-15.

Crespi, D., Mennini, T. & Gobbi, M. (1997). Carrier-dependent and Ca(2+)-dependent 5-HT and dopamine release induced by (+)-amphetamine, 3,4-methylendioxymethamphetamine, p-chloroamphetamine and (+)-fenfluramine. *Br. J. Pharmacol.*, 121:1735–1743.

Greer, G. & Tolbert, R. (1986). Subjective Reports of the Effects of MDMA in a Clinical Setting. *J. of Psychoactive Drugs*. 18(4): 319–327.

Johnson, M.W., Richards, W.A. & Griffiths, R.R. (2008). Human Hallucinogen Research: Guidelines for Safety. *J. Psychopharmacology*, 22(6): 621-632.

MAPS, Multidisciplinary Association for Psychedelic Studies, http://www.maps.org/research/.

Mintz, S. (2007). The War's Costs. *Digital History*. Retrieved 7/2/2012, http://www.digitalhistory.uh.edu/database/article_display.cfm?HHID=513

Mithoefer, M.C., Wagner, M.T., Mithoefer, A.T., Jerome, L. & Doblin, R. (2011). The safety and efficacy of ±3,4-methylenedioxymethamphetamine-assisted psychotherapy in subjects with chronic, treatment-resistant posttraumatic stress disorder: The first randomized controlled pilot study. *J. Psychopharmacology*, 25(4): 439-452.

National Institute on Drug Abuse.(2006). MDMA (Ecstasy) *Research Report Series*. [Electronic Version] http://nida.nih.gov/Research Reports/MDMA.

Parker, M.A., Marona-Lewicka, D., Kurrasch, S., Shulgin, A.T. & Nichols, D.E. (1998). Synthesis and Evaluation of Ring-Methylated Derivatives of 3,4-(Methylenedioxy)amphetamine (MDA). *J. Med. Chem.*, 41, 1001-1005.

Passie, T. (2010). Neurophysiological and Psychological Mechanisms of Entactogens in Psychotherapy. *MAPS: Psychedelic Science in the 21st Century, Conference*, April, 2010, San Jose, CA. http://vimeo.com/16704170.

Ricaurte, G.A, Martello, A.L., Katz, J.L. & Martello, M.B. (1992). Lasting effects of (+-)-3,4-methylenedioxymethamphetamine (MDMA) on central serotonergic neurons in nonhuman primates: neurochemical observations. *J. Pharmacol. Exp. Ther.*, 261(2):616-622.

Ricaurte, G.A., Yuan, J., Hatzidimitriou, G., Cord, B.J. & McCann, U.D. (2002). Severe dopaminergic neurotoxicity in primates after a common recreational dose regimen of MDMA ("Ecstasy"). *Science*, 27 September, 297: 2260-2263.

Ricaurte, G.A., Yuan, J., Hatzidimitriou, G., Cord, B.J. & McCann, U.D. (2003). Retraction of Ricaurte et al., *Science* 297 (5590) 2260-2263. *Science* 12 September, 301(5639): 1479.

Steele, T.D., McCann U.D. & Ricaurte, G.A. (1994). 3,4-methylenedioxymethamphetamine (MDMA, "Ecstasy"): pharmacology and toxicology in animals and humans. *Addiction*. 89(5):539-551.

Seymour, R. (1986). *MDMA* SF, CA: Haight-Ashbury Publications.

Foreword to the 2012 Edition

By Ralph Metzner, Ph.D.

Ecstasy... empathy...openness...compassion...peace...acceptance... being...forgiveness...healing...re-birth...unity...emotional bonding... caring...celebration...these are some of the terms people use to describe their experiences with a class of substances, of which MDMA 3,4-methylenedioxymethamphetamine (also known as Adam, ecstasy, Molly, or XTC) has become the best known. Although related in a general way to the psychedelic ("mind-manifesting") substances such as LSD, psilocybin and mescaline, these substances are different in that they do not usually produce visions, hallucinations, or altered perceptions of reality. Even more importantly, these substances seem to consistently induce positive affect and reduce or attenuate anxiety in significant contrast to the classical psychedelics which can amplify and elaborate both positive and negative affects. Because of the high percentage of major positive insight experiences reported with these substances, and the relatively low incidence of undesirable side-effects, these drugs have attracted favorable attention from a number of psychotherapists who regard them as facilitators of therapeutic insight and change. They have also been used by some teachers and practitioners of meditation who see them as important amplifiers of emotional and sensory awareness and as aids to spiritual practice.

The present book is a collection of personal accounts of these kinds of states of heightened awareness, particularly awareness of one's own emotions. They are remarkable both for the uniformity with which people affirm their positive value, and for the diversity and range of individual differences. The experiences reported here all occurred within a context of either psychotherapy, serious self-exploration, relationship communication, or spiritual practice. Some are accounts of individuals with psychological disturbances, including two rape victims who took the substance as part of their psychotherapy. Most of the individuals whose experiences are related here took the substances with guidance from someone experienced in their use in order to further their personal and spiritual growth.

The Use of MDMA in Overcoming Fear and Trauma

The book *Ecstasy: The Complete Guide*, edited by Julie Holland, M.D. (2001) offers a comprehensive look at the risks and benefits of MDMA, as well as summarizing the pharmacological effects identified thus far. Jessica Malberg and Katherine Bonson in their chapter on "How MDMA Works in the Brain," summarize the effects on the main brain neurotransmitters as follows:

> MDMA acts in the brain through three main neurochemical mechanisms: blockade of serotonin re-uptake, induction of serotonin release, and induction of dopamine release. With these actions, MDMA is essentially a combination of the effects of fluoxetine, a serotonin reuptake inhibitor and anti-depressant; a serotonin releaser and amphetamine, a dopamine releaser (Holland, 2001, p. 29).

More recent studies by Gillinder Bedi and others (2009) have used functional magnetic resonance imaging techniques to show that MDMA attenuated amygdala response to pictures of angry facial expressions, but did not affect amygdala response to fearful expressions. Responses to happy emotional expressions were enhanced with MDMA. Further studies done with recognition of emotions in facial expressions in photographs suggested to these authors (Bedi, et al., 2010) that MDMA reduced the perception of fear in the images, leading to more "pro-social behavior." Summaries and detailed descriptions of these and other studies may be found by consulting the MAPS website (www.maps.org), which maintains a comprehensive database of all published research on MDMA and other psychoactive drugs of potential value and interest.

These findings of reduced fear-perception are consistent with anecdotal reports (including many of those in this book) that MDMA significantly attenuates interpersonal fear and anxiety. This is probably the basis for its marked therapeutic utility, especially in the treatment of PTSD, where the perceptual fixations on a real life-threatening situation block the normal processing of memories.

The potential applications of MDMA in the treatment of debilitating post-traumatic stress disorder (PTSD), which is now being researched by Michael Mithoefer and associates at the University of North Carolina, is exemplified in two of the accounts in this book, whose authors were able to confront the traumatic experience of rape. One is called "I Can Now Move through the Trauma." She wrote:

> There seemed to be some quality of the Adam that broke down the repressive/defensive network and took me back into the experience of the attack that was too much for my psyche to bear. Over a period of eight to twelve months I was able to re-experience fragments of the attack, thereby recreating and de-sensitizing me to the experience (p.28).

The other account, by a school teacher, is titled "To Speak of What Was too Painful to Remember," and she writes about realizing that a rape that had occurred eight years ago, had been:

> [...] hidden in the back of my mind...and all the little details that I had wanted to ignore were eating at me like a cancer.... The suffering became more intense, but I still wanted to talk about it and I felt that I could deal with the pain, that this was a start to try to defeat this cancer (p.41).

The potential value of using MDMA in the treatment of PTSD can hardly be overestimated. There are some 350,000 veterans from US wars in Vietnam, Iraq, and Afghanistan who are suffering from PTSD (R. Doblin, personal communication, July 22, 2012) and who only receive palliative support, if any, from the usual prescriptions of SSRIs offered by the over-burdened Veterans' health care system.

One of the people I worked with in MDMA-supported psychotherapy in the early 1980s was a Vietnam war veteran, who was able to release an enormous amount of war-related trauma in one intensive session, and subsequently turned his life completely around, becoming a dedicated peace activist and co-founder of the group

Veterans for Peace, giving talks with fellow veterans on the realities of war to groups of high-school students (Ellis & Metzner, 2011).

A dramatic and powerful account of MDMA's ability to attenuate fear and terminal anxiety is given in the book by Marilyn Howell *Honor Thy Daughter*, also published by MAPS (2011). In this book, Howell relates how her 27-year old daughter who had colon cancer, struggled terribly to marshall her life-forces and resist the illness, in spite of the increasingly discouraging feedback from the medical professionals and increasingly painful side-effects of the chemotherapy drugs she was receiving. She fought for her life, using one extreme technological method after another. She didn't want to hear, think or talk about her possibly impending death. I think most researchers would agree that actually, for end-of-life palliative care the classical entheogens like LSD and psilocybin are better than MDMA at expanding awareness into the spiritual dimensions. But in the case of this young woman, since she was so relentlessly committed to fight for her life, and in denial about death, the turning point came when she could accept the possibility that the MDMA would ease her existing pain and anxiety, without thinking about death, the after-life or similar concerns. She was able to have a relatively peaceful and painless dying, in the company of her loved ones.

MDMA, Intimacy and Sexuality

Torsten Passie, M.D., a research psychiatrist at the University of Hanover Medical School in Germany, has done studies on the neurohormones released in the MDMA state and how this relates to the subjective effects. He states, on the basis of his studies, that MDMA deactivates the amygdala (the seat of fear-rage emotional reactivity) and reciprocally activates prefrontal brain circuits (which underlie calm thinking). This is the neurophysiological counterpart to the empathic understanding of self and others, reported by the patients. There is also a massive release of serotonin, the neurotransmitter associated with a non-depressive, non-fearful attitude.

Passie's research is described in a monograph published in 2012 by the Multi-disciplinary Association of Psychedelic Studies (MAPS) *Healing with Entactogens* by Torsten Passie, M.D.

To my mind the most provocative of his findings is that MDMA results in a massive release of prolactin, the hormone associated with breast-feeding, as well as oxytocin, sometimes called the "cuddle hormone." Both of these hormones are released during non-sexual post-orgasmic intimacy. As Dr. Passie points out, this release of non-sexual intimacy hormones correlates perfectly with the often-remarked subjective experience of MDMA-users—that they feel intimate with others, wanting to touch and be physically close, but not sexually aroused.

The experience of sensory and sensual intimacy without sexual activity or even desire is expressed in this book in the account titled "Desire Transcended by Being Fulfilled." In this account the subject, a 48-year old male, reported an experiment of having a massage at the Esalen retreat center, on two occasions—once without MDMA and once with. The man reported that the second massage:

> [...] seemed longer and slower, and my body responses much deeper and more total. I felt blissful. I recalled my wanting and desiring the masseuse, from the first session, and realized I did not have that craving or desire now; instead I felt as if we were making love! The desire was transcended by being fulfilled, virtually (p.103).

Even couples who were intimately involved have reported that with MDMA the sexual drive was often just not there. This effect is, in my opinion, one of the main reasons why MDMA has such unparalleled usefulness in enhancing psychotherapy. It facilitates the heart-felt, empathic, verbal and postural expression of emotional intimacy, without the slightest hint of sexual arousal or interest (which can be a confounding issue in therapist-patient interactions, as is well-known).

Entactogens vs. Empathogens

I want to say a word here about terminology. Torsten Passie, like most of the European researchers uses the word entactogen to describe the class of drugs like MDMA, whose primary neuropsychological action is a marked decrease of interpersonal and intrapsychic fear—thereby facilitating a seemingly effortless reintegration of previously defended and traumatic memories and perception. This is in marked contrast to the primary effect of the classical psychedelics (LSD, mescaline, psilocybin) which involve visual and affective amplification of all psychic contents and processes, including fear—thereby making difficult or "hellish" trips much more likely than with MDMA (where they are virtually absent). Entactogen means something like "touching within" or getting in touch with one's own inner processes.

In a friendly debate which I had with a couple of my colleagues in the pages of the MAPS bulletin several years ago, I suggested that "touching within" doesn't really distinguish the MDMA-type experience from the LSD-type experience. My own preferred term for these substances (and the experience they can facilitate) is "empathogen," generating a state of empathy, both empathy for others and empathy with one's own self in past or present conflict situations. This to me is the basis for the heightened affective understanding, the integration of emotion and reasoning, consequent upon the absence of fear and anxiety, that Dr. Passie's study (2012) demonstrates.

The Use of MDMA in Supportive Psychotherapy and Self-Exploration

When MDMA first became known in therapists' circles in the early 1970s, its possession or use was not illegal—until the FDA, invoking emergency powers, placed it on Schedule I in July 1985, just around the time the first edition of this book was published. Because of the change in its legal status, and for obvious reasons of confidentiality, the individuals reporting, the therapists or group leaders facilitating, and the researcher who compiled and edited the accounts all chose to remain anonymous. Now, more than 20 years later, MDMA is still illegal, and listed on the FDA's Schedule I (along with heroin, cocaine, LSD and marijuana) although researchers can obtain small amounts for their controlled and approved research studies. Such studies all have to be privately funded, since no pharmaceutical company can put its development resources behind it. In spite of the promising research studies demonstrating the relative safety of MDMA, and the positive anonymous self-reports published on the Erowid website (www.erowid.org)—MDMA is no closer to being formally and legally available for any condition or purpose than it was in the 1980s. However the informal, underground distribution of ecstasy at rave concerts, and in the context of small, anonymous, secretive groups, has led some observers to estimate (though of course no hard statistics are available) that several million doses of ecstasy are distributed and consumed every year—in the US, most European countries, as well as India, Japan, Australia, South Africa and possibly China.

The research with the classic psychedelic drugs (psilocybin, LSD, etc.) carried out during the 1960s led to the hypothesis, widely accepted by workers in the field, that psychedelics are non-specific psychic amplifiers, and that the content of a psychedelic experience is primarily a function of the "set" (expectations, intention, attitude, personality) and the "setting" (physical and social context, presence and attitude of others, including the guide). This set-and-setting hypothesis is also a useful model in coming to understand the experiences with MDMA. The specific insights, feelings and resolutions of problems that occur are of course unique to the individual, although there is a commonality in the kinds of feeling states that are named, such as "empathy," "ecstasy." Individuals are often able, if their intention in taking the substance is serious and therapeutic, to use the state to resolve long-standing intrapsychic conflicts or interpersonal problems in relationships. One therapist has estimated that in five hours of one MDMA session clients could activate and process psychic material that would normally require five months of weekly therapy sessions.

Because of the importance of the set and setting variables, a brief description of the nature of the set and the setting was requested of each of the individuals whose accounts were included. These are shown at the bottom of the first page of each account; and one can obtain a pretty clear sense of the operation of this principle by comparing that statement with the content of the experience. In addition, the text lists as "catalyst" the precise identity and the amount of the particular substance used. In many of the sessions, an initial dose was followed after an hour or so by a "booster" of a lesser amount of MDMA, or with a related compound called 2CB. Synthesized by Alexander Shulgin, the famous independent chemist who identified and synthesized hundreds of previously unknown psychoactive compounds (described in his books *TIHKAL* and *PIHKAL*), 2CB is in many ways analogous in its effects to MDMA, though much less research has been done on it, nor is it as widely available in the underground scene.

With all these empathogenic (or "entactogenic") substances, the catalyst triggers a change of feeling state, in which insights and perceptions take place. These insights and perceptions, though they may appear ordinary and commonplace when they are afterwards heard or read by others, are felt with a depth and poignancy of emotion that was for most people unheard of in their lives before the time of that first experience.

None of this is meant to say or imply that similar or identical changes of consciousness could not be produced or arrived at without the use of these empathogenic substances. Obviously, many people have in the past, and continue to have, empathic and heart-opening experiences without the use of any external aid, pharmaceutical or other. For the people whose experiences are recounted in this volume, the heightened and deepened state of awareness facilitated by the drug served as a kind of preview, as it were, a taste of the possibilities that exist for much greater emotional openness and relatedness than they had imagined.

They are clearly aware, too, that the drug-experience is a

temporary state, and one that can be converted into the ongoing reality of everyday consciousness only with continuing therapeutic and spiritual practice—and not with the continued use of the drug. Most people do not want to repeat the experience very often—it is felt to be too intense, too sacred. Although the possibility of becoming psychologically dependent on this, or any drug, cannot ever be ruled out, there is a fairly high degree of consensus that MDMA is not addicting, certainly not in the way that opiates are. None of this positive potential therapeutic work with MDMA discounts or denies the existence of patterns of extreme overuse of ecstasy that have become associated with the international rave culture, nor do we intend to minimize the potential harm from such overuse.

Under favorable circumstances and with a supportive set and setting people feel that the MDMA experience has elicited true compassion, forgiveness, and understanding for those with whom they have important relationships; and most importantly, for themselves, for their ordinary, neurotic, childish, struggling persona or ego. The relative absence or attenuation of normal amounts of anxiety and fear in these states is perhaps the single most important feature in regard to their therapeutic value. People report being able to think about, talk about, and deal with inner or outer issues that are otherwise always avoided because of the anxiety levels normally associated with those issues.

The accounts presented in this book derive from about fifty individuals, of various ages, professions, and degrees of psychospiritual sophistication. They were apparently gathered from about twenty anonymous therapists, mostly, though not exclusively, from the West Coast of the United States. Some of the reports are from guided therapeutic sessions; others are from sessions with serious psychological or spiritual intention, where the "sitter" might be a trusted friend or partner, rather than a therapist. A considerable number are by individuals who are themselves therapists—which suggests that some of the most promising potentials of these substances may lie in the training of therapists—where the capacity for empathy is highly-valued.

A smaller number of the reports are from group experiences, usually of a highly structured or ritualistic nature. Although the relatively unstructured, recreational use of ecstasy in informal small groups of friends is probably more common, most therapists are agreed that the use of rituals similar to those of the Native American Church, or other shamanic traditions, is the preferred mode of operation when powerful sacramental substances are taken in a group context.

The editor of this volume, the writers of the Preface, Foreword, and Guidelines, and the publishers, do not advocate the use of any illegal substance. Nor do they advocate that individuals attempt to treat their own medical or psychological problems with the use of these or any other substances. Nor do they recommend the use of these substances by individuals without the supervision and consultation of one's physician. Given these obvious limitations on the use and accessibility of these drugs, the question might be raised as to the point of publishing these accounts since MDMA is now illegal. The answer to this question, according to the therapists and their clients using these substances, is that it is in the public's interest to be aware of an extraordinarily promising new tool for the exploration of the human mind and for the improvement of human relations.

Perhaps greater public knowledge of these substances and their potential human benefits can lead to a considered re-examination of the social and legal framework with which our society deals with such matters, so that as other substances of similar import are discovered, their uses and potentials will not be wasted. Many of the individuals whose experiences are recounted in this volume expressed the wish and hope that, given the gravity of the planetary crisis in which we find ourselves, aids to the evolution of consciousness such as these substances will be thoroughly explored and applied to the solution of the immense human problems that confront us.

References for the Foreword

Ellis, E. & Metzner, R. (2011). From Traumatized Vet to Peacemaker Activist. *MAPS Bulletin*. Special Edition: Psychedelics & the Mind/Body Connection. Spring, (21)1.

Bedi, G., D. Psych., Phan, K.L., M.D., Angstadt, M., B.Sc./B.A. & de Wit, H., Ph.D. (2009). Effects of MDMA on sociability and neural response to social threat and social reward. *Psychopharmacology*, (Berl)., November; 207(1): 73–83. Published online, August 13. doi: 10.1007/s00213-009-1635-z.

Bedi, G., Hyman, D., de Wit, H. (2010). Is Ecstasy an 'Empathogen'? Effects of ±3,4-Methylenedioxymethamphetamine on Prosocial Feelings and Identification of Emotional States in Others. *Biological Psychiatry*, 68 (12): 1134. doi: 10.1016/j.biopsych.2010.08.003.

Holland, Julie (Editor). (2001). *Ecstasy: The Complete Guide*: A Comprehensive Look at the Risks and Benefits of MDMA. South Paris, ME: Park Street Press.

Howell, M. (2011). *Honor Thy Daughter*. Santa Cruz, CA: MAPS.

Passie, T. (2012). *Healing With Entactogens*. Santa Cruz, CA: MAPS.

Shulgin, Alexander & Shulgin, Ann. (1991). *Pihkal: A Chemical Love Story*. Berkeley, CA: Transform Press.

Shulgin, Alexander & Shulgin, Ann. (1997). *Tihkal: A Continuation*. Berkeley, CA: Transform Press.

Individual Experiences—Women

Earth Is Eden, and Adam Is Within

45 year-old female, teacher §

Ingestion of two white capsules at timed intervals...waiting...feel sensation of flotation and upliftment. Look at light fixture on ceiling...sudden rush of powerful energy and giant Presence; awed by the constant and immense sensation of an immovable force; choir of voices; the light fixture changes into a multi-layered mandala; face is a series of energy patterns shifting into varied mandalas of a kaleidoscopic nature....Realization that everything and everyone is a living mandala: awed by the experience; sensation of being within multi-layered patterns of energy that were constant change...constant change...but always beautiful, subtle, varied...simultaneously form, but not form.

Awareness that this must be what heaven is really like...see globe on table...'heaven on earth'...everything is on earth...heaven is on earth...moved by the wonder of it. No words in heaven...everything is beautiful, true, compassionate, loving, growing, changing, within this giant, constant, powerful presence. No words...too many needless words...power of the non-verbal touches me; I desire only to hum or listen to the grandeur of silence.

I am a giant, it is a giant; everything and everyone is a giant. My body is so small in comparison with what I am...tiny hands...tiny feet...just seems that way...a reminder of the power of the inner bodies; power of the spirit; power of formless form...great presence, beautiful spirit, eternal Immortal. Ancient hands, baby hands, giant hands... fascinated by my hands...feeling of giant walking within a doll's house. Sudden realization of the meaning of the 'genii' mythology...the lantern being the instrument of seemingly small vessel for the giant Spirit that is always within and a constant resource,

---

§ *Set*: exploratory, meditative.
Setting: friend's home, with guide.
Catalyst: 150 mg MDMA plus 50 mg MDMA.

guide, non-judging facilitator...constant presence, <u>immovable force.</u> <u>The term down-pour of energy has new meaning</u>...no words; just PRESENCE. I'm in heaven...wonderful, beautiful glorious heaven.

<u>HUM HUM HUM HUM HUM HUM HUM HUM HUM HUM HUM HUM</u>

Feel like hair is changing into feathers; hear hair growing; amazed at the civilization of vibrant life in my hair; hair changes again into feathers; feel a bird coming out of my head...<u>a hummingbird</u>. Thought: maybe my tumor was just a hummingbird waiting to be freed. Just then, he asks about my health...hear cracking of ice; something feels cracking in my legs; something pops in head. CONNECTIONS, connections.... Trying to take care of relatives, taken it all too far; take in too much; too extreme; too much the comforter, supporter, caretaker.... Disease with both extremities...leg, an extremity; head an extremity; hummingbird head; cracking-ice leg...polarities, opposites, dualities, paradoxes. TOO MUCH, TOO MUCH, TOO LONG. All not important, doesn't seem to matter...

what if everyone took this

no one would care

indifference

everything is all right

It's all a <u>theater</u>...it is all a <u>play</u>

If everyone took this; no one would care;

nothing would get done

because no one would care

Nothing important...always there is presence.

Purpose is not in the theater;

theater is not purpose

<u>What is purpose?</u>

Purpose is not tied to achievement;

purpose is not TIED to anything.

<u>Purpose is being like presence...</u>

<u>purpose is bringing light and love into</u>

<u>every situation</u>...with great PRESENCE.

Being present. New meaning for I'm here;

I am <u>present</u>. I am <u>a present</u>.

We are all presents; we are all presents!

Union, balance, absence of polarities...

absence and presence

Spirit never absent.

Decide that this is a good time to call up all my emotional images...one by one I select all the things that have activated me recently...reminded that it's all theater; can't get upset no matter how hard I try; state of great indifference. Images say what if B and F live together and have children...find myself happy that he's happy; feel close to him; great bond; deep love; great friend; can't get upset; what is there to be upset about; all ego and yet ego can't get upset; everything all right...we're great old friends; deep love; no reason to be upset; we love each other; no one can alter that; only add...everything adds; no anger; no betrayal; old patterns...no need to continue them. Amazed that I'm not getting upset...maybe I have worked through more than I thought...grateful, relieved, content, and great feeling of contentment, unflappability, objectivity...all of it just theater...no tragedies...just presence, light, power...presence, acceptance, compassion, trust...great friend—ancient love. Everything is all right. Can't get upset...such indifference from an objective place. Experience detachment...so this is detachment. Why have I been so upset in the past? Old patterns, old memories, old plays.

Strong sense that my head is expanding…feel like there's a small tree in my head. R must see the tree…I am a tree and he sees it. Tree in my head expands…branches in my head and arms; torso becomes trunk; legs and feet become roots. Legs/roots… tumor/legs/roots; branches/head/tumor…leg/roots…head/branches…combination of old/roots and new/branches…attempting to integrate old and new; ancient and modem; past and present. I'm in a season…no, two seasons at once: Spring and Fall…growing and letting go simultaneously.

HUM HUM HUM HUM HUM HUM HUM HUM HUM HUM HUM HUM
>accept

>>acceptance

>>>no problems

>>>>everyone is a tree

>>>>>everything is theater

>>>>>>different acts

>>>>>>>different seasons

>no exceptions

>only acceptance!

>No words

>Be present…original present

Take this perspective with you…just be an objective observer with all of my presence. Embarrassed by how much power I have given to what doesn't really matter. Re-focus, re-align, re-adjust back to Self. Image of dragon going to chiropractor flashes before me; I was born in the year of Dragon. Inner chiropractor is aligning the central axis and my inner levels or bodies fall into place. Smiling Dragon.

Look at my arms, hear the hair growing on my head; skin filled with copper...copper swirls; close eyes...cells, organs, centers, everything filled with copper patterns and spirals...everything is copper. Taste metal...strong metallic taste; is this the mineral kingdom in the body?...Beautiful, luxurious copper. Magnificent.

HUM HUM HUM HUM HUM HUM HUM HUM HUM HUM HUM HUM

Life, civilizations in the body...alive, vibrant, copper! healing copper...feel warm currents of energy; melting sensation; fire...small fires in the body; bonfires...feel like a furnace. Dragon furnace; Copper Dragon...fire breathing Dragon! Solar Plexus furnace...copper furnace...the solar plexus is a copper furnace. Healing furnace...healing copper.

It's all theater...I sat under a tree with a Genii who released the hummingbird that sang to the Dragon in the Doll's house that was made from copper. Everything is a mandala, and heaven is on earth. Great presents on earth: purpose, presence, acceptance, and love. Earth is Eden, and Adam is within.

HUM HUM HUM <u>HUMBLED</u>

I Was Resting in the Palm of His Hand

35 year-old former school teacher, ex-nun §

Perhaps the most obvious feeling for me at the beginning and throughout the session was the incredible sense of peace and release from the bondage that I felt. My body was no longer a trap, a prison, but instead became like a kaleidoscope, a mingling of different energies. I felt myself being several "I"s in a very strange way. Sometimes I felt myself very wise, sometimes I was the adult me (not so wise) and sometimes I was a child. I felt a deep friendship with the guide, as if I had known him for a long time. Certain other relationships came up and I saw them as equally lovable. I was able to detach from intense attachments that bring pain and was able to love gently and freely, a truly wonderful gift for me.

I found myself thinking of God the Father and felt that I was resting in the palm of His hand, just as Isaiah says in the Bible. I was being rocked in a large hand with darkness as universe all around me. It was incredibly soothing and loving. When the guide put on certain music, I felt romantic, and instead of being with God the Father, I was dancing with a very handsome man whom I don't know. It was very peaceful, not passionate; very graceful and free. Then I was confused, and it became the figure of Jesus. I was amazed. I told the guide that Jesus was my brother whom I loved very deeply. The guide suggested that Jesus was also my lover and yes, I have felt that, though a bit guiltily. But love like that with a man is what I have sought…passion and gentleness together…peace. In my life both aspects have always been separate. A man is either passionate or gentle, and I love both, but they are separate.

I knew instantly what my life's purpose was…to continue to seek the heart and mind union, to continue to remember the essence within which was so peaceful, in spite of worldly activities. Adam revealed

---

§ *Set*: therapeutic, spiritual.
Setting: therapist's office, with guide.
Catalyst: 150 mg MDMA plus 50 mg MDMA.

a new potential which I knew was there, but was too afraid to experience alone. As far as my studies, I realized they were important, but they only mattered in the world. I saw that I was worrying too much about others' opinions of my work. I realized that the intellectual work has been a saving grace for me...I truly love the work of the mind, I have always been an avid reader. But, now I can put it in perspective. I have been putting too much energy in concepts and theories that may change in ten years, whereas the eternal principles of love, truth, self-realization, etc., remain the same. Now I can, with the help of Adam, tap into the deeper resources which were always my goal. I am still a bit afraid of the future, of going back "into the world," but after the session, I feel that the inner connection will guide me through and I will find my place. The place will definitely be working directly with love energies.

When the guide played Vangelis' *Odes* I felt as if my soul had been called. I remembered my Greek heritage and I went back to ancient times in feeling and memory. I felt very, very old. I could have died at that point and not felt bad about leaving my loved ones. Somehow I felt that they would understand. Death was so natural, so peaceful.

With the South American jungle music, I felt very earthy and that felt threatening. I felt that I was going to be sacrificed, and my dream of running away over the mountain was remembered. Going into instinctual waters is very scary for me, I realized then. I felt the possibility of the mind gone wild, of no principles to live by, of evil sorcery and of life being worthless. Since then I have realized that I feel the same way about certain areas of the ghetto where I grew up. in fact, some were even called "the jungle." There is a sense of being ripped open and apart. I have felt that passion does that, when it is purely egotistical desire without taking the beauty and dignity of the human being into account. In some ways, my quest for the spiritual was to purify myself from those threats. I have never seen that before. But I think I definitely have to face those instincts now, though I am afraid.

During the session I saw my mother's life and realized that her suffering was hers, not mine. This has been a great release for me. I saw that, just as I could have died then and there and known it was right, that she also, at some level, perhaps had that feeling. I could see under the normal layers, in a way, and know that we all know the truth underneath. So too my mother may have known that someday I would understand and accept her death, without feelings of abandonment. This was a wonderful gift. When I thought of my father, I missed that sense of security and power that comes from the male (at least for me) but I was getting it from God the Father as energy and love. I was able to see my parents as earthly extensions of Divine parents and as such of course limited. But since I now felt the presence of Divine parents, it was O.K. I still hold that feeling to this day, though not as strongly as during the session.

I realized that I have a hard time receiving love, I mean, really experiencing it. I know that I am loved, but I feel shy and don't seem to give it much importance. I felt a deep sense of self-love, a feeling of rightness about me, as I was. In loving freely, I want to give without expectations but also receive without judgment. I see this very clearly. It will be my life's goal. I'm really excited about it. Life now becomes a mystery, but a good one. Before, it was always a problem. As a mystery, I am not judged if I am me, I am looking to see who that "me" is. And looking, in itself, is worthwhile. Another relief.

One of the most beautiful experiences of the session was the resolution of Christian and Buddhist compassion. This has been an inner question for me for many years. How could Buddha love and not feel sad; how could Jesus feel sad in loving and still be enlightened? Somehow, during the session, they came together. I saw that Jesus's heart, sad with the ignorance of the world, was an expression of his life externally, but that internally, he was absolutely sure that he and the Father were one and so, his soul was at peace. Buddha's external expression was mind, a peaceful, harmonious mind, but his internal experience was a deep sadness and heartfelt compassion for the suffering of the world. So he, too, gave his life to save others from suffering. For me, Jesus and Buddha, in front of whom I pray and meditate, became two sides of the same coin, two perspectives of one experience. That question is over and I am truly grateful, for I can cultivate both heart and mind, knowing that sadness and peace can be simultaneous emotions or feelings, and not judge them as separate. Also, that sadness and love are one aspect and that joy and love are also expressions of love. Love can and should also be practical.

The 1000 Petal Lotus Unfolding and Unfolding

45 year-old female, housewife, mother §

Why did I want to take Adam?

I have been feeling an emptiness inside—a loss of meaning for my life. I visualize myself as a crysalis—something is dissolving and something is reforming. But I do not know the shape of what is there—I am not in touch with my Essential Self. I want to find my spiritual connections—the sound and taste of my own Emerging Self. My outside persona is still pretty intact, pretty recognizable, but there are profound physiological and psychological changes happening as I move from being a fertile woman and a wife and mother to being an Older Woman alone. I want to accept the changes with more serenity and inner joy.

So I am asking my Self how I can best come to some acceptance of my life as it is today? Where do I find the courage to make the further changes that are necessary and to let go of the rest of the stuff that is no longer relevant? Where are the rose-colored glasses to change my attitude so that I can truly enjoy the freedom of living alone? How can I best achieve the serenity to take each day as it comes and not try to recreate the past or worry about the future?

How can I open my heart again? I feel so shut off from Love. I feel afraid to be loving and light-hearted and foolishly affectionate with anything or anyone. I want to reconnect with that innocent, joyful part of my Self.

Yesterday my guide gave me a great gift of Adam. It took about forty-five minutes for the drug to take effect, so we sat in the living room and talked together. It was so lovely just being with her.

We started with music of Kitaro. I drifted a while. Then I began to see amazing patterns. I had thought that there was a void but it was so complex and intricate...wonderful. I thought about trying to

---

§ *Set*: self-exploration, spiritual.
Setting: home, with guide/friend.
Catalyst: 150 mg MDMA plus 50 mg MDMA.

capture them and paint them or reproduce them, but I knew that I did not want to do that. I could not hold onto them—I just had to let them be and enjoy them. Some of the patterns were like feathers—peacock feathers and pheasant feathers. I felt like the designs were a message to my Self—that there is all this complexity—that life is very rich.

Then there was star music—very swooping. I saw a great tree against the sky with dragons at the ends of the branches and milkweed against a blue October sky—cranes flying and great blue herons. I felt as if I were flying. My legs tensed and my shoulders and my back arched and my jaw tightened. I felt as if I were poised to fly.

I realized that I do not have to do anything different with my life. It's all here now. I don't have to change my life. It is very full now! That feels good to me!

The essence of this experience for me was a deeper Knowing. I did not hear voices or see psychedelic pictures with colored shimmering edges. I seemed to tune into a source of strength and knowledge that has always been there but that I have forgotten. I "saw" with new clarity and without sentimentality.

I checked in with some of the people I love. I thought a lot about Love, that there is love all around us, that there is lots of love in my life and I haven't given enough credence to all that. All these people I have been checking in with love me and I love them. I found that I don't know if I really want another marriage partner—or even a sexual partner—that I don't want to do trips with people, that I am afraid to put the effort required into making another marriage, that I want someone to play with and to have fun with—but that there are lots of loving people in my life already.

I saw a far-off bright field with sunlight shining on it and a path leading away from some gates and over a hill. I saw some men walking away from me down the path and over the hill out of sight. I realized that is probably true—that there are not going to be any more men in my life, at least as a real partner. Then the gates swung closed. However there are lots of people in my life and I don't need a man. I don't need anyone else. And someone may come, but I don't need him. It is the sense of neediness that is so awful.

Beautiful flute music, skimming over the California landscape, appreciating how beautiful the world is. Then I came to some wide adobe steps leading upwards in a slow spiral with a flat building at the top. The whole structure seemed to be turning around a fixed axis—the North Star. This is the experience of the Divine for me—I am a humanist—I don't need a supernatural god. There is so much beauty all around—and so much love—and so many wonderful people. That is enough. I feel very open and I have felt so closed off and unloveable for so long. I feel that this is a process of polishing the glasses and seeing what is there.

Then I got something about Trust—I got that you can trust other people to live their own lives, that I don't have to mother people anymore or take care of them. I know that my task now is to work on myself and to find my own strength, that I don't need the other person anymore. I feel that I have connected deeply with a source of Strength. I didn't hear any words and I didn't see very many pictures, but there was a deep KNOWING that I could connect with. I feel wonderful about myself—I don't have to try so hard. Just to be! Simplify things a bit and spend more time with myself.

During this experience I had various body sensations—I felt very light most of the time except for the muscle contractions that were not all that distracting—added to the sensation of flying. I checked throughout my body and I feel very healthy—no pains or aches or problems. My body is serving me well.

I checked around to see if there was anything that I could discard in my life, any way that I could simplify things. Actually there isn't very much that I want to give up. But I could go more slowly. All the people in my life are very important to me and I cannot stop seeing any of them. But I have to clearer about how much space I need for myself. I want to stay connected with all the people I love, and I know that staying connected takes work and time and loving energy and I have lots of that loving energy now. But I know that people will respect my need for more space and it will be easier for everyone if they don't perceive me as being so needy.

More lovely peaceful flute music that sounded like wind—like the breath of God—and I really came to know that there is Spirit all around us. I experienced the 1000 petal lotus unfolding and unfolding and unfolding and I knew that you can never really get to the Center—but that it is there!

We talked again about Love and my feeling so shut off from it. This whole experience has been an Opening of the Heart. I want to move through each day more slowly—being here now—not quite so frantically, not in such a panic about being left alone. I want to enjoy my solitude. I saw that this could be a time to make some commitments that would serve to keep me in this space of Inner Peace of Heart.

I am just starting out on a Path and I don't know what is going to happen, but I want to allow whatever is going to happen to happen.

After the experience I felt incredibly high and relaxed and happy, but the next day I started to come down and felt so exhausted that I began to question the whole experience. Did I really tap some Inner Truth or was this all a clever pre-programming by the music and the discussions that we had while the drug was entering my blood stream?

For a few days I was unsure about accepting any of the Wisdom I had touched. Then I realized that what I had experienced was an enlarging of my reality, that the Truth I had seen was only a part of a larger whole and that there was even more—and that it was all true. That ended my doubting and made it easier for me to integrate the experience into my everyday relationships.

I decided to secure the experience by making some changes in my life. I decided that I wanted to begin to meditate regularly every day again, and I have been doing that since day 4. That has been very calming and has helped me get back to the peaceful space that I experienced with the drug. I decided to listen to music more regularly—just listen to music, and not use it as background, but listen with my heart and that, too, is wonderful.

About day 8 I realized that I knew what Unconditional Love means! I feel this great gently loving feeling—it doesn't require doing anything—I don't have to earn love from anyone by doing something for them. I can just be there with them and love them and with most people that is wonderful. I got lots of positive feedback from the other participants in my graduate school.

Now I feel easier with all the people that I love—fewer obligations and neediness. I feel that I have dropped my concerns for their happiness, that I can trust them to find their own way. This is an extension of my growing awareness that I am through mothering other people—I am finally ready to focus on mothering ME.

It is now two weeks since my Adam experience. I am sleeping much better—no aids for 4 nights. Mostly I am feeling calmer and more at peace with the universe than I have for years. I made a couple of lovely monoprints to illuminate Rumi's poem:

> The clear bead at the center changes everything
> There are no edges to my loving now.

It is still difficult for me to accept the truth of my knowing—so much of my everyday reality seems contradictory. I am beginning to accept the paradoxes.

The Energy Flows Through Me, I Make It into Music

35 year-old female,
graduate student, computer programmer §

Since I've found a place where I can bridge my higher self and my ego, I don't have to live trapped in my ego. I don't have to be trapped in the hurting part. That's hopeful, that means that we humans can be something more than the evil part of human and it also means we don't have to become Jesus Christ to do it; it's not such a big mountain to climb. We can heal ourselves without climbing to the very heights; there is an in-between place that's reachable for all of us. So that makes me hopeful. At the same time, when I see something like *The Killing Fields*, it makes me so overwhelmed with the feeling that the job is so big, that there are so many people, the majority that are trapped in that other part and don't know about the god within. And what those two things, those two extremes, the hope and the sadness/desperation about the world, make me feel that there is something I need to do more than just work on myself. I need to help heal the world. And I don't know how to do it.

It's something more than just being kind and a teacher to the people who work for me, because I feel like the problem is so overwhelming. The problem is so overwhelming, yet there's the hopeful part that there is this place. If I can be here—and when I say "be here" I don't mean just here living in my Christ consciousness, I mean be here pissed off, and all of it, I mean be here all of me, yet not let the part that separates and destroys control me; if I can do it, then the next person can do it.

We're working to get to the place where we can step aside of our egos and be in the place of love. The pain is still there, it's not denied, it's felt, but there's another avenue we can use, and the pain gets healed. So, I need to do the healing in my life, that's where I work

---

§ *Set*: exploratory, therapeutic.
Setting: at home with partner, friend sitting.
Catalyst: 150 mg MDMA.

first. But, now I can feel 'cause I don't feel so much a captive of my own problems, 'cause I feel those are workable, I feel it's not enough to just do it in that little circle that I do it in. I've always seen the need for the healing but I never saw that there was really an out, 'cause I was also a captive of my ego, but now I've watched how in the last several years I can get out from under that control.... I've always felt the pain of humanity, but now I see that there is hope, that if I can do this then others can. So, that's the change.... The change is not that the pain of humanity has lessened; there's been a ray of light in all that pain, and the ray of light is "I am able to step out of it."

I find that the Adam experience now tends not to be so distinct from the rest of my life, it starts to be part of life without taking anything.

My body does not exist from my hips down, but my back right now feels like it is absolutely on fire! Oh my god, my back is burning up. It's going up to my head, too. Is this what they mean by kundalini? It's incredible. It's like you're on fire. Incredible! I've had it in the lower back before, but this is up into my head. Lot of it around the higher back, the heart.... I'm staying in my body 'cause this heat on my back is keeping me more in my body. I guess that's my lesson, to stay in my body more. It's this heat. I feel like I'm going to be sick to my stomach. It's burning up. It's in my head burning up too.... This heat is keeping me in my body. I also feel sick to my stomach. There are flashes of white light again. I see, I've been working on bridging there and here: the heat keeps me in my body but the light can still be here. Last time I got lost in the light, this time it just comes and goes. The heat is burning up, going up out of the top of my head. I'm shaking. It's burning, burning. I feel like my head is on fire. It started on my lower back, but now it's moved up my back, and in my head. It's like it's on fire. Incredible. The light peeks in now and then. It's as if something else has overtaken my body.... Amazing.... My mouth is so dry, everything is burning up. I can't swallow, it won't go down.... It's just this heat moving up my back. Now it's at the base of my neck between my shoulders. It flows up into my head. Part of me is outside watching it. I felt no fear, no resistance or dread, etc.

The white light isn't steady this time.... I really am learning all the time. I'm not getting any messages this time.... Now the heat seems more even up and down my spine.... Now it feels like it's spread in my whole back.... There's heat everywhere.... With the heat here I'm staying in my body. I guess that's what I want to do, bridge all this, bring it together.... My whole body is vibrating.... I just had a vision of the world as a person, the same separateness from self as a person....

I'm very much here, I'm not out of my body at all. The music makes me see little people living in harmony.... The music is playing my brain.... It's burning around my heart.... I feel like having energy in my heart but I have to move it out so it can come back.... I don't know if this always happens, 'cause I'm usually not in my body, but my mouth is like a desert! It's like the energy is forcing itself out of my mouth now.... Energy....

Rushes of energy go through me, waves of energy, and I shake (waves of shudders from my toes to my head). It's rushing up my spine to my brain.... This energy is incredible. It's in waves. Going in waves clear up me.... I give myself very little space to be...to be and not to try.... This is my lesson, to experience all this in my body.... I already know the learning. I just need to go with what I know....

Waves of energy are going through my body. Incredible.... It's like I'm a clarinet, and you blow on the clarinet and your breath comes out the other end but so does this wonderful music. The energy flows through me and what I can do is make it into music; it doesn't have to come out of me the same way it went through me. I can make it what I want, but once it leaves me there can be music that goes with it, so the next person it hits, it's not just energy (breath), it's also music. I always felt that because it has to be channeled through my ego, it would lose its music, but that's not true. Sometimes it does, sometimes the ego can be pretty dense and dark. My ego is the clarinet. I feel like I'm completing the bridging of ego and Self. Something happened here. Oh, the light just came on; I guess its affirming that something happened. The ego is the clarinet, but the higher Self is the musician. Yes, that's it. So, not only does energy not have to be stuck, but it doesn't have to come out as just energy, it can be music. I want it to be love.

Springs of Enchantment

26 year-old female, student §

I discovered Adam when I started an affair with this psychologist, who was using it in therapy. I broke off with my boyfriend, from whom I felt estranged and distant, even though he was very hurt and convinced that we were meant for each other. My sexual feelings became reawakened, after a long slumber.

A few weeks later I moved to a holistic health retreat in the country, where I obtained a job, and began to study hypnosis. My former boyfriend was also there. I didn't want anything to do with him at first, even though he was very needy. Then after a while I thought it would be good if we took Adam—maybe it would help him and it would make it easier for both of us to accept our separateness.

During the session we became very close again, and I saw how he was right: we really were supposed to be together, and learn to work together. So we fell in love again. I called the psychologist friend, who was expecting to see me again, and I told him what had happened. Now he felt hurt and rejected.

He said the Adam experience reminded him of the enchanted springs in the magical forests of Arthurian legend. There was a spring, according to this legend, such that if you went there and drank from it you would fall asleep, and when you woke up, you would fall in love with the first person you saw. There was also another enchanted spring nearby, with the opposite effect: if you drank from it you would fall asleep, and when you woke up, you would fall out of love with whomever you were infatuated with at the time.

---

§ *Set*: relationship communication and bonding.
Setting: outside in nature, with partner.
Catalyst: 100 mg MDMA plus 50 mg MDMA.

All of Me, Just Being

42 year-old housewife, mother §

Here I go, plunging forward through something I don't really like to do—and yet I know with surety how important it is for me to look at where there is resistance.

I felt extremely peaceful, all of me just being with whatever came up—a real lack of self-consciousness. I liked being so completely that way. Gentle. Slow. It was a gift to myself being that way. It was also a gift being with my wonderful friend that way. I trusted that I could be me.

I liked having the eye shades on. I liked going in. As soon as it was on I was reminded of my first acid trip when I closed my eyes and <u>wouldn't</u> open them for a long time. On acid I had sunk into my grief over my dead son. This time I started to cry, and I felt wonderful crying. I felt my guide might stop me from crying so I said that I was fine, that I felt good, that I needed to do this, that I felt in touch this way, and that it has been a long time. It was wonderful being together with him.

I loved the music right off. I just went away on it—expansive. I wanted music that I could go along with. I just lay until I was moved to speak—slowly. I liked going at that pace. I'd love to always move and be that way. It was good for me to experience myself that way. A good reminder. I've intentionally slowed myself a number of times since then, in acts like brushing my teeth, doing little regular acts. I realize I hurry and there's a level of tension. Then I catch myself and take better care of myself, slow down, and feel great that I did that.

I remember feeling that my life felt very much in order for the most part. I feel like acknowledging some people, like Werner Erhard— really for his level of going for it.

I felt very loving. Also with my mother, which is not an easy

---

§ *Set*: self-exploratory.
Setting: home, with guide.
Catalyst: 150 mg MDMA plus 50 mg MDMA.

relationship. I genuinely wanted to hear how and what she felt about hunger, nuclear issues, and like that. I was aware that I just wanted to hear without judging or making her wrong, that I could hear whatever she had to say without there being any tension in my body. I felt very good about that, Dear Mom!

I held my face between my hands as if I were someone else, my lover, holding it. It was a very interesting and enjoyable experience. It felt so small to me. (People have always said that I have a small face).

I remember being overwhelmed by the incredibleness of this planet and really wanting people to stop and get it. Then there wouldn't be even the possibility of destroying it.

I remember my teeth really chattering. I've never experienced that before. I liked it. I could stop it. I did want to be in control!

My picture of myself is changing. Let through the new me— whatever that happens to be at any given moment. I feel I need to meditate and I intend to make that a part of my daily life again. I've done a number of the items I said I would already. I feel good doing what I said I'd like to. I feel powerful making it happen.

To Bathe the World in Light

35 year-old female, graduate student §

How do I help my ego to not be afraid? I'm not in the fear right now. The ego is afraid of me "dying." What is so funny is that I'm fearing something that's already happened. It's like fearing that your house is going to burn down when it's already burned down. I'm afraid of…. Last time the fear was that I would leave my body and that I would die. But it was my body that was afraid. I want to stay here a bit to work with this, it's starting to make some sense. The fear is silly…but the ego will take over…that ego of mine is really feisty, she wants everything, she wants it all for herself.

The ego wants everything, it's like an octopus grabbing and grabbing. Ego wants to control and it gets threatened. The reason my ego is so threatened is because I've lived so much of my life not here. The ego knows it has a very tenuous hold. Meditation threatens my ego, all my spiritual work threatens my ego. So, my ego tries to take hold of it as its own. "I'll be more perfect and more spiritual," that's the ego. What the ego has to know is that the change in me is that I want to integrate, to incarnate, I want to be here, the ego does not have to be threatened. I realize for the first time that I want to be here. Being here is being there. When I go out there I'm not in my ego anymore and my ego needs to hear this, I need to stay with my ego so my ego can know this. I'm not my ego…my ego is that little pea, my ego is a part of who I am but I am not my ego. My ego is a subset, just a little pea.

I have been living with my mystic self as my dominant self, and my ego is threatened, is not sure that I want to stay here, so of course it gets terrors. Since my ego sees that the mystic is where I'm at, it wants to take on that, so it says "Okay, now I'll be a mystic" and in order to be a mystic it must be perfect. So it, the critical self, is trying

---

§ *Set*: exploratory, therapeutic.
Setting: at home, with husband and friend/sitter.
Catalyst: 150 mg MDMA.

to be a god; that's it, if it can be a god it won't be threatened. It's like this piece of clothing is trying to be the body, trying to be my heart. So that's why I'm always beating myself up for not being perfect. That doesn't make sense but I just know it, I know it's my ego trying to be god.

And another thing, if it could just relax, it's already happened. It's all already happened! My ego is trying to be the boss, and the critical self is a tool for it, it is grasping at being the master, it can't stand that it's not the master. The message to the ego is that I do want to live in this world, when my body is ready to die it will die on its own, I am not going to leave the ego. I want to be here, I've never been able to say that before. Marrying was one step to making a commitment to being here; letting myself get close to some people was laying the groundwork to making the commitment. I do want to be here. I've lived a lot of my life going away, in a trance. I do want to be here.

Now let's get to the fear. What I fear is death, but I'm fearing what is already there. Who dies? It's my ego that's scared. When I go away, it's just nothing but a feeling in my heart when I come back. And there's a feeling that I did not die, that the nothing was something. But, there are no words for it. I see blackness, but black has a connotation of...it's just the heart, just the heart. It's not empty, it's the heart. No, it's not nothing because everything's there. It's not empty, it's not anything that I can tell. My body's going away again; I'll hold your hand to stay grounded here. It is love. When you come back, this is what you bring back. And it feels so wonderful. I want to feel this way always.

I'm seeing just white light, but it's not...I just got scared. My body is very sensitive, I think. I just saw bright white light, as if my eyeshades were off. My ego is becoming scared. If I let go I just go, I don't trust that I'll comeback.... This is just gorgeous.... I left my body again, the way I know is that I am looking at my body breathing. It's on automatic pilot. It breathes, I don't do it. It's safe out there but my body gets scared that I won't come back.

The light...even though I have eyeshades on it's as if the sun with all it's power is shining...it's this white light that is shining. It's just this shining in my head, shining! It's like everything is just white light. My eyes are closed, eyeshades are on but it just shines. There it goes into my heart. Now I'll focus it in my heart. It's just light! God! Last journey there was just nothingness, now there's still no visual images, just light, white light. Oh God! Oh my! It's as if...I don't know what it's as if...white light. Incredible. I don't have a tense jaw. My body is...it's hard to get it back, it's very little, a little gossamer body. Oh there's the white light. Oh my God! Oh my God!.... I'll send it to my heart.... No wonder my ego is so threatened.... Sure is a lot of light out here.... I'm going away for awhile into the light.... Oh God!.... God...it is just light. Incredible. Oh...it's bathing my whole body.... The light is always there, it's a matter of whether I'm open to it. Like the heart, it's always there. It's a matter of whether I'm open to it. We are there, we are that heart.... Nothing new to report in here, just a lot of light. Nothing much is happening out here! (Laugh) I'm in here, the light follows me into my body.

I think I'll come back to my body for a bit, to check in. I went away for awhile. My body just drops off, there's no body anymore, then just light. Oh boy! I want light to go everywhere in the world, to bathe everyone, to bathe the world. The fear is that little ego. Initially I was afraid of the light. Poor thing, she's had such a tenuous hold. The light is like grace, it's just there bathing you. I don't feel like it's something I can control.

I've been having a feeling that I know what grace means. It's nothing...it's like a washing that I can't control. Opening up. When the ego sets out to be perfect, there's no grace. When you get away from that (ego), and just open up, something wonderful happens.

I don't have to go away from my body to be with my mind. I can experience it here with my ego. My ego needs to know that this experience does not deny the ego. The ego sees it as either/or. It's duality. The ego really can't see beyond duality. It's part of the whole but it can't see that; I can see that....

I can see myself breathing. I no longer feel the breathing but I can hear it—I guess I hear it. I'm watching this body here breathing but I am in no way connected with the breathing. Like, I got a twitch in my leg, but it goes on without me. When I'm far away I don't feel the twitches or hear the breathing, but as I'm just leaving I get the sensation that it's all going on without me, that I'm watching this happen to a body, but it's not...I don't mean it's like a near-death experience, but that somehow I'm separate, watching it happen. I'm totally dissociated.... The feeling of the heart isn't as strong this time, it's there in wanting to bathe the whole world. It's like a prism, the same experience with a different angle on it.

The white light is more...I want to say impersonal...there's a feeling that I want to bathe everyone, but it's different from the heart. The white light is...transpersonal, yes, that's what I'm tying to say. I think the heart is, too, but the heart comes through something. That's the difference, the heart goes through emotions, but the light doesn't go through emotions. They're both beyond the personal, but...it's just so unpredictable. You don't have to go away to have this, it's all here; this ego that is so threatened is sitting in the midst of it already. It's OK for the ego to cry, to get disappointed, and all those things. That's what the ego <u>does</u>. So, the ego gets hurt, that's what the ego does. It's okay. It's just the ego getting hurt, that's all it is. The ego is all these little people, and it's very self-critical.

I go out and come back in with it. I seem to be able to come and go better this time. The going got so that it wasn't frightening at all. So maybe I should look at that in terms of letting go of a lot of things. It's the ego that won't let go, that is threatened.

We have details that are different but there is still the essential sameness. All these egos, God.... The me behind the ego has no little parts. The ego is little parts, no real one identity, but here there is a single...being—I'll use the word being. It's like all the egos are made out of the same recipe; there are different proportions but its all made from the same ingredients. There's nothing that's unique, and the ego works so hard to be unique—an illusion.

So just feel the heart and say, "Oh yes, that's the ego; she wants to be perfect right now, she wants to be loved. She's loved." They're like little children—they need to be cared for like children. But it's true that we're so much the same. What an amazing thing! I think I've known this. When I feel love for someone I feel it by seeing that.

To release the hold of my ego, which is threatened and holds on so tight, is to be more fully here with it. It's the paradox that says the more I become it the less it will be. By accepting it, it can let go a bit.

The feeling of opening or closing—in the body, too—is the love coming or not coming through. Let the ego be with the knowledge of the vast room, let it just be the little pea. It's not getting <u>rid</u> of anger or fear, 'cause that's what the ego does. So, let the ego do all of its things but from the perspective of the vast room. It's okay to be angry, it's all okay. And we all do it. We really are everybody. That little ego that has been kicked around is everybody's ego. The uniqueness is to me my ego, but if I step out of the ego and look around, then this ego is not unique. Only the proportions of this ego are unique.

We are all the same and so much energy is spent denying that. When I say I know someone's experience, I'm coming from my heart, from that part in me that is like that part in him. There's no part that he has that I don't have in some proportion. He doesn't understand when he's coming from the unique ego-identification level. Part of the lesson for me is to discover the sameness. When someone fucks up, I find that endearing. I need to remember to apply that to myself. It's so touching to see all of our egos struggling—your pain is my pain. That's how we know each other, because we are all the same....

When I went out I felt like all I had was two huge hands. We exist on a lot of levels.

I saw the light again. Last time I came back feeling how the god within us is all the same, but this time it's the egos, too.... Acceptance is the key.

I Can Now Move Through the Trauma

35 year-old female, therapist, rape victim §

Here is a general account of the effect that Adam had in the aftermath of the attack I experienced.

I suffered from some memory block or repression around the specific events during the attack, which has prevented any cathartic work. All of the terror has remained locked up inside of me and I have felt stuck, afraid—and victimized by everyday circumstances in that I have had flashbacks of sorts: everyday sights, sounds, <u>anything</u> (a particular noise in a restaurant, someone walking up behind me, etc.). Things that I was not consciously aware of would trigger the unconscious nightmare that would result in dissociative responses that polarized and terrorized me.

There seemed to be some quality of the Adam that broke down the repressive/defensive network and took me back into the experience of the attack that was too much for my psyche to bear. Over a period of eight to twelve months I was able to re-experience fragments of the attack, thereby re-creating and de-sensitizing me to the experience. During the Adam I moved in and out of the attack: being plunged into the horror, then moving into a transitional phase of regression, into what was reported to me to be an almost infantile state (for example, during my re-experience of the attack my hands were either immobilized or assumed protective movements; after the horror the hands would gradually switch to small, infantile movements). I was not conscious of this phase. I was also told that I would often move into a fetal position and at times I would make slight, involuntary sucking movements.

My experience seemed to alternate between these two phases, and at times I would "come around" with what was reported as an exceptional presence—a vibrancy and change in color—an expansive

---

§ *Set*: therapeutic, integration of traumatic experience.
Setting: therapist's office.
Catalyst: 150 mg MDMA plus 50 mg MDMA; 4 sessions over 12 month period.

quality rather than a fearful, contracted quality, and with a beaming sort of aura. I _felt_ expansive, physically exhausted, but full of love and a deep feeling of peace. It has seemed that the Adam has allowed me to move into the fragments of the attack, to re-experience what I have needed to re-experience, and to desensitize me to my surroundings. The dissociative episodes have ended, and I can now move through trauma and come out of it in an open, loving way rather than leaving me with more memory of assault.

I want to clarify one further point. I had no conscious choice about the first part of the trip, in which I relived the attack, even when I _tried_ consciously to maintain contact with my sitter. I would lapse back into the event and eventually regain focused, conscious awareness. I would phase in and out of the attack five or six times within a three to five-hour period. It was most intense during the first two hours, when it was clear to those who were with me that I was horrified and in great pain. It was from these episodes that the event was reconstructed for use by the police. It was as though I had been transported into a trance-like state. I often did not remember what I had blurted out and this was later fed back to me for integration. Throughout this past year I have been experiencing violent nightmares, waking up soaking wet, not remembering much of the content, so that the nightmare state and the Adam state were somewhat similar.

Affirming Who I Am, Where I Am Going

37 year-old female,
graduate student, systems designer §

Whatever I can say now only dimly reflects my meeting with myself under Adam's influence. These phrases and ideas from the transcript remind me of some of the highlights:

> There's an opening that wasn't there before....

> It's clear that everything I'm about, and
> everybody is about, is just loving God,
> and how to do that...

> Guide: Does this remind you of your previous
> psychedelic experience?

> Answer: This is quite different. Much more
> important. Much more personal, much
> more relevant. Much easier to carry back
> and to apply. I've got so much love and
> compassion that attaches itself to
> anything in the vicinity and tries to make
> it seem appropriate. That's when I forget
> that what I'm all about is loving God—
> then I try to put too much into any
> relationship.

> There are still levels of integration to do
> around sexuality.... There's a real confusion
> of some kind, ...a real split.... Now I'm

---

§ *Set*: self-exploratory, meditative.
Setting: at home, with therapist/guide.
Catalyst: 150 mg MDMA plus 50 mg MDMA.

listening to my inner voice—usually I tend
to avoid it.... Sex can be a way to get closer
to God, but I haven't been choosing in such
a fashion that it's going to be.... It's been
very helpful to be celibate because I can see
so much more clearly and easily where my
sexual energy goes, where my attractions are.

What is the source of my arthritis?
Blocked energies. I need to get in touch
with what I want, and let the knowledge
lubricate my joints: no more stoppage
of anger or love. Let it all flow through!

Guide: So love lubricates the joints!

Material about a sexual molestation incident—first reported during
a hypnosis session several weeks ago—has had much more meaning
for me since I heard the tape of the Adam session. In it I sounded like
I was seven years old. The impact comes from the deep recognition
of how many ways the event molded my responses to the world
around me, in part because of the distrust of my parents that was
focused by the incident. Reliving this incident helped to free up my
energy and emotions in a number of ways; it feels like this process
will be ongoing for some time to come. The understanding and
resolving of this incident is not only helpful to me personally; it can
be a vehicle for my reaching out to others with similar experiences.

In general, my journey with Adam affirmed who I am, what I am
doing, where I am going. The affirmation was experienced through
an opening of my heart rather than as a deepening of intellectual
understanding, although some of that has also occurred.

The Adam, the set, the setting, and the invaluable input and
support of the therapist/guide created a sense of receptivity, wonder,
love, and joy. In this set and setting, with empathy for all aspects of

life, learning took place whose content was easily and deeply received. My desire to access such learning is great, in part because recalling these lessons elicits the highly desirable state of consciousness in which the learning occurred. The content itself also seems to take on a certain desirability, making it more readily available than much that I have learned under more traditional circumstances. Just writing about the state now, almost a week later, still brings back the sense of wonder, love, and joy that I felt at the time.

My mind tends to scurry about, trying to give form to some of the issues that were raised on the trip, but which still seem incomplete. These include a deeper understanding of my confusion about/dissatisfaction with past relationships, sexual matters, use of alcohol, and future plans for my internship, dissertation, and profession. Despite the attention that these topics get, I am for the most part holding them lightly: I have a clear sense that my journey with Adam is far from over: much is being considered and reflected upon below the surface of my conscious awareness. To the extent that I have addressed these concerns I am very well satisfied with the understandings I have reached.

My actions as well as my attitudes have begun to shift in certain areas. I am able to perceive, receive, and respond to love in a much more open way than I did a few weeks ago. There is a greater ease with respect to my dealing with and responding to my sexual energy. I seem to find it much easier to contact my feelings and, as appropriate, to express them.

Perhaps the most important after-effect has been the indwellling experience of affirmation about what I am doing. There is a sense of correctness; even when feeling muddled and unclear about what is happening, I know at a very deep level that I am moving in the right direction. However dark the path, however many shadows may appear, there is a light within me that provides warmth, illumination, and nourishment. My awareness of this indwelling light and my increased clarity of my sense of purpose has been greatly enhanced by my experience with Adam.

The Fire of Love and Trust
Banishing Demons of Fear and Pain

32 year-old female, psychologist §

I thought often of my breathing, wanting to focus on it because of my problem with asthma. I felt disembodied—it was hard to tell whether I was breathing or whether my heart was beating. I would draw in my breath consciously—not knowing how long it had been since I last did that. At one point I worried that I would have to go to the hospital because I had stopped breathing. I decided that if that happened that I could handle it. There was no experience of fear.

My lover asked me to consider whether I had asked myself the question, "Do I deserve love?" I had never considered it in that way before. I realized that I wasn't sure. I experienced strong somatic effects when considering this idea, feelings of contraction in my gut. Not unpleasant. I began to feel that my breathing problems were connected with my fear of "doing the wrong thing," which would lead to loss of love.

I realize that fear permeates my life, veritably smothering me. My lover told me he loved me for who I was, not what I did. Somehow this thought brought sadness. I had the thought quite a few times that there must be some reason other than me, myself, that I was loved—for example it was karma, or that I was loved in spite of myself.

I began to have strong waves of feeling blessed, that I was incredibly fortunate to do the sessions, to be able to open up my heart and mind and look inside without the usual barrier of fear.

Post-session realizations:

The fire of love and trust will banish the demons of fear and pain. I had very old, childhood pain of abandonment by my father. The

---

§ *Set*: therapeutic, self-exploratory.
Setting: at home, with partner as sitter.
Catalyst: 150 mg MDMA plus 100 mg ketamine simultaneously

worst part was not knowing what had happened, and never seeing him again. I have had no trust that any man that I love would stay. I feel that I'm easily forgotten. I feel bad that my father forgot all about me. I realized that my father left because he was unhappy. I did not do anything to cause that. I did not create it, Mom did not create it; if anything Mom and Dad together co-created the problem. They both were doing what they thought was best. Dad probably thought that it was better for the kids if he did not come and visit. I forgave him for making this mistake. I forgave Mom for what she did and for not explaining.

I usually fear that abandonment will happen with the man I love, that he will find someone with whom he would rather be than me. I experience this pain and fear when he doesn't call when he said he would, or when I can't find him. I fear that, like my father, I will never see him again.

I am now sure that the man I live with will continue to exist when I don't see him or hear from him. I now know that we have a special connection that will never be broken, even after we die.

A Secret of Life Revealed

48 year-old female, artist, mother of two §

We finally found a night for the Adam experience. In no time I was carried into a different state of consciousness, very hard to put into words, certainly very different from an LSD experience. The main difference for me was that an LSD trip brings about a lot of mind-images, it seems—there is more mind expansion or explosion; whereas Adam brings about this intrinsic, unique sensation of body-awareness where one floats in total bliss. This sensation of blissful floating was shown in my mind as energy-forming, expanding, contracting, breathing (one could say: breath as moving and life-giving)—each slight movement creating a minute change in the energy field, made of what we call "love" in it's purest and truest form of existence. It was truly mind-blowing, awesome, a secret of life revealed. This most unbelievable gentleness and sweetness we are! Thank you so much for this beautiful gift. There has been nothing like it, so real and so long-lasting (about nine hours), before in my life.

The sweetest sounds come out of me, following the movement of my outbreath. Again and again. So gentle. Such full and expanded in-and-outbreaths. When I threw up, it was just like that, nothing but a natural action. It's true, though, that in the beginning, when it hit me, my partner took care of me beautifully, moving me from one place to the other. He felt me to be three times as heavy, whereas inside I felt light as light and without any resistance or weight, with only the sensation of my body giving me a natural feeling of boundaries.

Also, all levels of consciousness seemed to have slowed down tremendously and to have become one—no separation whatsoever, inner and outer as one, no mental thought interfering, just communicating the experience of the moment, in a sense no past, no future, all simultaneously happening at once. Soul-talk. So simple, so

---

§ *Set*: exploratory, relationship communication.
Setting: at home, with partner also on trip.
Catalyst: 300 mg MDMA.

beautiful, so poetic. My partner and I experienced each other in the fullest soul-sense. Whatever we would be doing—talking, moving, looking, making love, being, it was real as real as anyone can be. It was so easy to understand one another, so true, gentle, blissful.

What joy! I couldn't believe how simple life really is. If we didn't have our beliefs and thought-forms blocking us, we would constantly be in a state of fulfillment. Somehow the "I" (whatever it is—it seemed full and empty at the same time) knew at every instant what it wanted or needed and expressed it, clearly and simply, with the sweetest voice and without hesitation, distrust, or disconnectedness. The "I" (Self) was just love and the mind served it most beautifully with clear, simple words.

Love is truly beyond words, and because it exists, everything else is created with it and through it. The question of the Will came up for me: who is willing here? Certainly it is not my personal will. If it is the universal will, or whatever, it's hard not to interfere with it through personal distortions in our normal state of consciousness. What an art it is to live life happily, creatively, with fulfillment Most of all I want to remember how simple life really is.

Clairvoyance and a Sense of Open Truth

48 year-old female, artist §

Having taken Adam only a few times, my experiences have nevertheless been varied. I had no drugs previous to this year. During the first session I experienced myself as a cross of light and my arms automatically spread out, whereby a great clearing in the body-emotions-mind came about. This first session was in a natural surround, and trees were seen simultaneously as trees and as energy fields and temples. Clarity and direct cognition about aspects of my life that were previously dimly felt occurred. Flashes of insight touching all 48 years of my life came, whereby consciousness went down through fields of awareness that might be called past-life resonances, even to the point of my entry into the earth for the first time in the Himalayas, when I could change my body into light waves.

During this clearing and purification, whole processions of memories of people went by whereby I felt great gratitude and spontaneously felt a warm-hearted bestowal of blessings to others. Although I had no intention beyond open experiencing in this first session, it answered many questions. I was told that it would be a three or four-hour session, but after some time I discovered that it was not the sun in mid-heaven but the moon, for the sun had set long before and it was midnight! Over twelve hours had passed.

With two subsequent sessions I had specific questions that I wished to be instructed on, and I found that if the mind is focused on an inquiry or is open to some truth, insights concerning the issue are revealed, consistently.

One thing that I am most impressed with is that the insights about my life and about the lives of others are so profound that I am motivated to immediately take action. This has turned out to be very

§ *Set*: exploratory.
Setting: outside, nature.
Catalyst: 150 mg MDMA.

effective in my daily life. After the first session I cleaned up my whole garage (which literally had four tons of stuff in it). After the second I gave dietary and exercise instructions to my mother, who had been suffering for many years from severe arthritic pains and problems due to her being overweight. Not only did she respond to my instructions (by mail, yet!), but she is no longer in pain, and the signs of arthritis have miraculously lifted. She has lost considerable weight and feels more positive and clear and happy in mind.

I suspect that Adam experiences are quite unique and custom-made to the individual. Motivation, integrity, and the degree one has prepared one's life for true insights make, I feel, a lot of difference in the kind of experience that one has. I feet that I have no need for repeated sessions, at least for the present, for the clairvoyance and a sense of open truth in expression that it has helped to open continue for me as a sustained way of life.

Such Deep Compassion, Such True Caring

39 year-old female, filmmaker §

The first physical sign of the drug became evident about an hour after taking it, when I felt my hands to be "airy," as if they wanted to just gently fly off on their own. Simultaneously, something that was said touched me deeply, and I felt very emotional. There were, however, few similarities with psychedelics. Adam is much gentler, and there were no visual hallucinations. There was a distinct emotional effect. I felt that my most compassionate aspect was in full control. I was able to see and understand other peoples' actions from a totally neutral place, with a compassionate feeling for them, even if their actions caused me pain.

I had access to feelings of love, compassion, and forgiveness for my father. We have had a lifetime of difficulty in our relationship, and since he is very old and sick I have been troubled lately that perhaps he might die soon without ever having experienced a good communication between us. This experience assisted me in seeing him and his situation in a very giving, caring way, and to let the difficult aspects of our relationship fall away. It was a totally new feeling for me that I had never had for him before, and it was a healing experience for me, and, I hope, for him.

The drug seemed to bring out my gentlest, most compassionate nature and to suppress the more judgmental, critical aspects of my personality. These are definitely part of my make-up, but are not the parts of myself that I am most proud of. It was actually quite lovely to feel such deep compassion, such true caring, to such a great degree. It was a very genuine feeling, and I could see why people had spoken of this drug as one that could enhance relationships.

But it was also much more. It provided an ability to see clearly, and, as my guide had told me, to access information from what I call

---

§ *Set*: exploratory, therapeutic.
Setting: at home, with friend as sitter/guide.
Catalyst: 150 mg MDMA.

universal consciousness. It could also foster intuition and encourage the flow of creative ideas. Most of the time I was lying on my bed, listening to music, going deep within to ask questions and receive answers. Occasionally my guide would comment, or offer me water, or turn on the tape recorder when I wanted to tape a thought or idea.

I felt, and still feel, an enormous love for her, and a great appreciation for her gentle guidance and caring for me. She made sure that all of my physical needs were met, provided the most perfect music I could imagine, and generally was 100% there for me in anything I needed.

At one point, since I and others are working on a project about US/USSR citizen diplomacy, and are concerned with peace issues, my guide asked me to look and see what impressions I got about where the nuclear threat was going. Were we destined to blow ourselves up or was this increasing nuclear threat just aberrant behavior that had gone too far off balance? It felt as though this nuclear threat we are experiencing is some sort of test, a difficulty placed in our path for us to overcome. I asked other questions and received answers, all of which seemed familiar, as if some part of me already knew these answers and needed only to be reminded of them.

One thing is certain: I'd like to be able to access these feelings of compassion and deep caring in a selfless manner at other times, and so I am working on remembering this feeling and am keeping connected with it. The entire experience was very valuable.

To Speak of What Was Too Painful to Remember

26 year-old female, school teacher, rape victim §

My perception was very keen. I seemed to be a lot more aware of the moment. Like the first time there was a flowing of emotions and I started to cry. My friends' presence gave me reassurance and I was able to trust myself to go deeper into my past and speak of painful aspects of my life. I knew that my friends were there to help me and I felt the need to pour out my agony. My emotions were becoming too much to handle, they seemed to be poisoning my veins.

By this time I was too scared to keep going deeper into my past. My friend asked me to keep silent for ten minutes and to think of and feel what was happening to me. It took a long time before I could do this, always fearing that I would simply go mad. When I finally accepted it and did it, I could feel the pain take over my body so that the suffering was physical as well. I was alone in this suffering. I felt that I had to go through it, if I was to accomplish anything. This was an important challenge because after ten minutes of too much pain I was able to trust myself to speak of what was once too painful to remember.

I spoke of a rape that occurred eight years ago. For eight years I have kept the most horrible aspects of that day hidden in the back of my mind, and it was only then that I realized how the little details that I had wanted to ignore were eating at me like a cancer. The memories became very vivid in my mind and the suffering became more intense, but I still wanted to talk about it and I felt that I could deal with the pain, that it was a start to try to defeat the cancer. Adam made it possible for me to speak and to try to see things from a different view.

By talking about it I was able to face the fear of the experience and to understand what it had done to my life. It was frightening to think that I had tried to ignore that day to the point where I didn't

---

§ *Set*: therapeutic, integrating past trauma.
Setting: home, with friends/guides.
Catalyst: 65 mg MDMA two hours after 300 μg LSD.

know where the pain had come from, nor could I remember what had happened. I had gone through life having nightmares and feeling guilty, telling myself that it was not normal to be affected by something that has occurred such a long time ago.

The most destructive feeling that resulted from the rape was a feeling of inner emptiness: I didn't feel love or hate for the people who had hurt me; I didn't feel anything toward myself and even less for life itself. (This is the reason why I don't like anti-depressant drugs: they make me feel the same way.) I continued living because I didn't even care enough to kill myself. I remember crossing the street and thinking, "If a car hits me, fine, and if it doesn't, that's fine, too." It's much worse to not feel anything even than to feel something sad.

So my emotions caught up with me, and I was closer to death than I'd ever been before.

Adam has helped me look at this suffering, to see my life as a whole and to understand it better. It has given me the courage to face the fears instead of ignoring them, to know that the most important thing is to struggle to trust myself. I don't know what my life will be like now, or how much I want to live, but I do know that the experiences I have gone through, even though painful, have also been full of tenderness and trust, and there is no longer this feeling of emptiness. I am not leaving a hospital with a prescription in my hand for anti-depressants. Rather, I'm leaving with a friend, with the hope that I see him again, and with the courage to try to face my fears and to face life.

It has been the vision of so many deaths, during the LSD portion of this experience, that is helping me to live now.

About two hours after taking the LSD, my friend asked me whether I wanted to take Adam. At this point I would have tried anything, and I thought that the Adam would help me cope with this pain, so I said yes. It didn't ease the pain but it helped to open up the emotions that were bottled up inside. Once I opened to my memory of the past, the room seemed to fill up with people from my past who had hurt me, and with people who had tried to help me. My friend's eyes seemed to be calling out to me, but then all of a sudden he changed and became transformed into the rapist. His toes and legs were those of the rapist but I knew that the figure was my friend. It was horrifying to see him as the man who had caused me so much pain. The only reason I could deal with it was because my friend was so strong in being himself that even though his body seemed to be that of the rapist, the rapist could not take over his mind, and I could turn to him for support.

I started to feel the horror of that day and I started vomiting. Getting sick was more than just a physical illness. I was vomiting from my soul, getting rid of pain, of an evil that had been destroying me. I felt then the need to tell my friend what the rapist had done to me, having always kept it to myself because I thought that by not speaking about it that eventually it would be erased from reality, and that all of it would become a horrible dream, a part of my imagination.

I felt that it was too late to pretend that it hadn't been real, and I feared that my friend would hate me. I don't know why, maybe it was that I hated my own body, it being a reminder of evil and corruption. But he didn't feel disgust towards my body, he didn't see it as changed by the experience. I then tried to see my body through his eyes, to understand that it was not impure, that it didn't have to be a reminder of cruelty.

I felt that I was becoming stronger with my friend's help. The rapist was grabbing me inside and wouldn't let go. I wanted to vomit so badly, feeling that if I did I could be rid of the rapist—at least he would be outside and no longer a part of me.

Later I felt I had got rid of so much, but I still felt nauseous, there was still a burning lump in my stomach. But no matter how hard I tried I couldn't get it out. It seemed to be the only part of the rapist that remained. Maybe it will always be there and I will have to learn to live with it. But it doesn't have to dominate my life.

My physical discomfort interfered with the peaceful movements that were also a part of this experience. They seemed trivial compared with the pain, but now I hold them close to me and they help me cope.

I felt that it was so painful to love that knowing that I could still love was what caused most of my suffering. But the emptiness and pain of not loving was so much greater—without love we cannot experience the beauty of living. I felt that I had to hold on to the love instead of fighting it, and that I had to try to deal with the pain that it caused me, because facing it is better than the emptiness.

It seems hard to do, but perhaps there is a chance that I can fill the emptiness with new life. It scares me and I feel very lonely. But this experience has made me realize that death is not necessarily the right answer, or the most peaceful alternative. Realizing this has given me the courage to at least try to find meaning and reason.

The Chooser Becomes the Chosen

45 year-old female, artist-filmmaker, mother of two §

I lie back and listen to music, feeling pulled to touch my heart (chest) with my hand. My hands begin dancelike movements in the air and suddenly I am hit, full front, with a chemical buzz and I see exquisite patterns of colored energy dancing against a dark background. I sense this energy, which will go <u>wherever</u> it is directed, it is indifferent to the outcome of what it serves.

It speaks to me: "The experiment is (essentially) over." I felt a wave of anguish and I prepare for sadness. It speaks again: "There's no sadness." I feel confusion. I report aloud, "There's no sadness." My guide speaks: "Not after a while." From him I feel compassion for us all....

I close my eyes again, to go beyond "energy." I feel (even now as I report) a deepening recognition of the larger picture: that there are "levels" or "states" at which it matters a great deal and there exists a vast well of feeling, but that the energy itself does indeed not care. But for the earth itself, and for that which created it there will be grief that I cannot yet even begin to fathom, of gigantic proportion. I am reminded by my guide that we are indeed more than earthlings.

I am guided to allow myself to accept that creation, at least the human family, may be destroyed. Humans will, in this scenario, destroy themselves. This is a real (and perhaps realistic) possibility. Yet, in accepting this, I see a path which branches off from this field of acceptance. And so we come to the beginning of the path I am now on: "God, grant me the courage to change that which I can change, the serenity to accept that which I cannot change, and the wisdom to know the difference." This feels like Phase I.

The next phase begins with a sense of "What can I do?" The guide

---

§ *Set*: spiritual exploration, self-healing.
Setting: at home, with friend/guide.
Catalyst: 150 mg MDMA plus 50 mg MDMA.

clarifies that through acceptance I can lessen the grief of the impact of future outcomes. I can have a say in what happens by transforming my acceptance into an affirmation.

With great tenderness, the guide puts his hand on my heart center, leaves it resting there, and asks "How is your body?" He reminds me that this is an opportunity to heal the spirit AND mind AND body split—not just mind/spirit or spirit/body or mind/body....

At that point I become aware that what I can do about the larger situation is allow, invite, surrender God into my own body. The God consciousness aches for and eagerly awaits this moment to enter me, as it longs to enter each of us, at any and every moment. I lay back and turn my palms upward. Without resistance I say "I sacrifice myself. Who is there? It is I. Who is there? It is I. Who is there? It is Thou."

Painlessly, and in silent ecstasy, that which has lived as my guest, my visitor, my "higher" self becomes part of my consciousness. We merge. No longer higher, it is now inner, merging with that which chose. The chooser becomes the chosen. The guide knows. He speaks of gods and goddesses with open eyes all over their bodies. Phase II ends here, with the glad marriage of myself and my Self.

In the third phase, I begin to relate this state to daily reality. Others. The network. Cultivate the network. Adam simply turns up the volume. It is all already so. I review my life from this heightened awareness. What is acceptable? Unsuitable?

My physical disorder—I search inward and discover resistance to the physical plane. My guide encourages me to observe patterns in Nature and give birth to creative patterns of order. The phrase "the order that enables us" helps free my thinking. I remind myself that if I am becoming a home to the indwelling spirit, it will see out of my eyes, and it likes to see beauty, proportion, and harmony!

I realize that I can make agreements with myself in the Adam state, that I can recall them when in the non-Adam state, and that can affect the non-Adam state. I proceed to ask for guidance and support in integrating these changes of habit into my life. I do intend to become a perfect temple for this God-consciousness. I plant the seeds of support in myself this day. Another agreement I make with myself is to let it shine, not to hide or be shy about this energy of the spirit that is infusing me.

Phase III continues in daily awareness, acknowledging what is unacceptable, and, with compassion, designing ways to clear the core—yes, like a reed flute, so that the breath can pass through and be, if appropriate, music. Phase II continues also, since I choose and rechoose every day. And I dwell in Phase I, the acceptance of that-which-l-cannot-change and from which action springs,,

Final phase: manifest, receive, accept, create, share, allow, generate <u>LOVE</u>, It is the gravitational force of and for the spirit.

I had always felt unconscious of and therefore cut off from my own body. It's as if the part of me that lived such a full life was a visitor, who took no responsibility for the house in which it stays.

During the course of a single Adam session, I experienced a deep natural healing within myself. I re-owned my body. In the two weeks that have followed, I have observed specific behavioral changes in myself. These include: the ease with which I choose lighter, healthful foods, and no longer desire heavy, fatty foods; a definite increase in the grace with which I move; an instinctive desire for water with a marked increase in daily fluid intake; no desire for caffeine or alcohol. And for the first time in my life, I can feel myself consciously and lovingly aware of the body in which I live.

Body/Mind/Spirit Move into Hovering Space

37 year-old female psychologist, healer §

Question posed: I feel a natural evolution of love, integrity, creativity, and power. What is my way to right action in balancing the personal and transpersonal dimensions?

Body: a feeling of evenness. Calm anticipation. Then contraction and expansion. Imagery: a flower and a stone. I'm falling through space. My left side is a large stone out of which an enormous flower blooms on the right side. The flower acts like a parachute.

Body: warmth starting up legs through pelvic bowl. Imagery: I am the earth. Body feels as long as the earth. Head is the North Pole. Sun shines and warms entire body except North Pole (head). Does the earth feel this too?

(Music: "Timewind," by Klaus Schulze.) Image of wind whipping around me. Cutting through something on the diagonal. Feel like a mummy being unwrapped. Body energy and awareness increase.

Suddenly a huge trumpet flower emerges out of the equator of my earth body (navel) and reaches up far into space.

Wind sounds feel cool and draw my attention to the North Pole. Ice and snow. Energy forms that look like transparent comets whirl around at high speed. They have a numinous quality. Raindrops form from these energy-entities. Fall to earth and become crystals in a cavern in the earth.

I am aware that life is formed in the wind. These energy forms feel like basic life (breath). They seem to be Spirit, travelling at high speed. This Spirit is apparently the essential truth that we experience once we leave our bodies. This Spirit appears to be what energy is between lives: invisible, yet, in a numinous way, present.

I asked my guide to read the "Emerald Tablet" of Hermes Trismegistos:

---

§ *Set*: spiritual exploration, planetary consciousness.
Setting: at home, with friend/guide.
Catalyst: 150 mg MDMA plus 50 mg MDMA.

"...The father thereof is the Sun;

the mother is the moon;

it was carried in the womb by the Wind;

the Earth is the nurse.

It is the father of all works of wonder throughout

the world."

Little wind spirit relaxes and becomes a raindrop. Raindrop falls to earth, slows down in this touching, and becomes crystal. Shifting vibrational speed manifests all things.

The guide suggests that I tune into the earth's axis. When I do, I feel the earth's etheric bodies. Body/Mind/ Spirit move into hovering space. I refocus on the floor of the crystal cavern at the North Pole.

Clear and definite image and feeling of an Animal Spirit to my upper right. A black panther encased in sandstone, Egyptian stone guardian, sitting proudly, with dignity. There is a certain stillness in that dark power. The guide suggests the stone image is just one manifestation: "Look into its essence." I see the stone outer cat serves as a container, a cocoon. This reminds me of my own body, and though it serves as a vessel for Spirit, it's important to watch for rigidity and fixed notions and viewpoints. Stone statue's name is I-You, which speaks of this ego-skin between self and other. On the other hand, the essential life inside this skin speaks of being true, direct, moving with spontaneity and unselfconscious passion.

The guide suggests I move inside form. My body experiences heavier energy coming in on the right side. My guide invites my feminine side to open to receive.

Image of a black warrior with a rainbow extending out of his head, starting to enter my body on the right side. Feels like too much power. Immediately an image emerges of a black man and a white lotus. This white lotus fills my vision. It is incredibly beautiful, with 1000 petals. It floats over a pool of water, never stopping. It is rootless, yet it is sustained by something. The image evokes a quality of the Form and Formless. I later see that its roots are grounded in the Formless.

I look at a picture of a strong black woman, well grounded and balanced. She has a lithe, solid body, and is wearing a lavender dress. Her face is hidden behind a crystal veil. She stands in the rain near a lagoon. In her hands is a large straw broom, and she seems to be sweeping with much determination.

I experience a deep sense of integration, feminine strength, and fullness. Lavender is the color of a warrior. The contrasting colors of black and lavender represent to me the dense and the subtle. I feel enlivened and awake and right when I look at this picture, because it is a way of synthesizing the male and female energies. The panther and black warrior energies are incorporated in a form that fits for me. The act of sweeping is a metaphor for a style of clearing in my healing work: caring, cleansing, clearing.

Image of mouth flying open: awe, shock, no sound. I have no idea where this image/sensation comes from. Image of me as a baby in a crib, my cries unanswered. Feeling alone. Strong impression of being outdoors under an enormous black sky, experiencing vast space and distance from the shimmering stars. Alone, crying out into vast emptiness.

On the psychodynamic level, from the feeling of aloneness, I developed an attitude of "I'll do it myself. I won't let you help me. I'll take care of myself, because I know you need a mother more than me. I'm more in touch with my own wisdom."

Developing a stance of independence. Giving more than receiving. I see that I continually need to practice reaching out and asking for what I need. The reaching out is definitely harder for me. Aware of being more a rock in the stream, defined by many who want something from me. I am practicing being the stream and flowing and reaching for those I want to be with.

I become aware of tension in back of neck and along jawbones. Holding back and controlling my responses. Seems to be some psychodynamic clearing. Some question about fear of sexual surrender. Although I've opened to a far deeper place of surrender at this point, there is past memory of confusion and fear. Not deep sexual fear, but rather confusion about being seen as too powerful to be given to (as a healer), yet seeing myself to be in part a needing woman.

My guide asks "Are not both true?" Yes. My concern: if I surrender sexually, or if I fall in love, I fear I will lose my power. I saw my needing as vulnerability and weakness. In the past this has been true. I still need to clear past conditioning on this. I'm caught in a collective feminine notion about giving over to a man, which doesn't seem to further relationships in the 80s. How sex role behavior patterns hold on!

The guide suggests a redefinition of the feminine/receptive to include reaching out. Simple sentences, such as "I need you to be with me and share sexually. I want to be with you. I want time and space to enjoy you. These are my needs and wants...", etc. Bringing these essential things into my being brings me into balance and harmony. This, for me, is a bowing in respect to all chakra energies, and acknowledging that all are open, are functioning correctly.

The day following the Adam session, I worked with my therapist to see more deeply into the nature of the crying baby. Uncovered an incident with my mother which cleared easily. Found an earlier incident related to birth trauma of being born feet first and almost suffocating as head came through the birth canal. Experienced blank space/black space, something I've never felt before.... Seems linked with anesthesia given to my mother, combined with her fear of death. Apparently Adam kicked off a sensation of this. This work is in progress.

An incredibly fine experience for me on many levels. R, your willingness to guide me through this touched me. The direct experience of Energy, Life, the Earth, first human life, the 1000 petal lotus is precious to me. The images are rich and clear. The assimilation and reintegration of male-female, animal-flower symbols and emotions is an empowering experience for me. I am surprised the psychodynamics all poured out. So be it.

Out of Nowhere Appeared My Inner Guides

40 year-old female, therapist, mother of three §

This is a report on my first Adam session. In preparation for the session I cleaned my house. I sensed that this was going to be a sacred experience, and I wanted to prepare myself in a sacred manner. My guide came, and we went over a list of questions I had prepared to focus on during this journey. My guide suggested an additional question for my inner guides or higher self: "For my highest and best good, is there anything else I should be aware of at this time?"

I put on an eye-shade and listened to music. Time passed quickly; I felt the loving support of my guide, and then I started to feel my body having sensations I have always associated with excitement. Then out of nowhere appeared my own inner guides. They moved out of a gray fog, and for the first time I felt no fear of them. Always in my meditations I had been afraid that I was going crazy when they tried to speak to me, so I stopped meditating.

There were about ten of them, dressed in draped gray garments, and I could tell by feeling that some were male and some were female. They felt like my real family. They spoke to me, not in words, but in mind to mind communication, about the importance of meditation for my growth. They said I was afraid of meditating because I had not learned to ground myself adequately, and that I must practice grounding meditations for a period of at least a month. They said to imagine myself buried in dirt, to meditate from this position, and to be sure that I used grounding tools during therapy. All my fear vanished.

The next question that was dealt with was my issue with weight. My guides were not present visibly, but information came into me: it is not food that I am craving, but liquid. I had misread my body's signals. I should be drinking a mixture of warm water, warm milk,

---

§ *Set*: self-exploration, therapeutic.
Setting: at home, with therapist/guide.
Catalyst: 150 mg MDMA plus 50 mg MDMA.

and honey to lose weight. It was very important to lose weight so I could resonate with a different frequency of energy. Too much flesh was preventing this process from taking place.

There followed a period in which a lot of information came to me concerning new inventions. One related to a metal box that contained particles; a laser gun was attached to it. People would be connected to it with wires, and their thoughts would be transmitted to the box where they would be transformed by the laser gun into a language read by a computer. Next there was information about pesticides and insects. The chemicals that we are using now are too heavy; a new family of non-toxic light chemicals that man will be able to live with will be invented. Insects should be sprayed with substances that make them feel love and acceptance: then people will live in harmony with them.

A question about my son was dealt with. My guides told me it was necessary for my son to go and live with his father. I was very sad, but felt it was all for the best. I cried a lot about my son during the session. I felt that I was being pulled apart. After my boyfriend came over to take care of me, and my guide left, I experienced a deep love and bonding with my son. I felt such love for the gift he has given me.

My question about why angry men are attracted to me was also answered: they want my warm loving-mother energy they didn't get when they were young. Later in the relationship, all of their anger at their mothers comes up and is directed at me.

I was very emotional all night long. I cried a lot for all little children, for how painful and confusing it is for them and for adults. The next day my friend took me to a beautiful location overlooking the ocean. I was very moved by Nature, more than I can remember being since I was a child. I could feel and sense the presence of the Miwok Indians, and how blessed they had been to live in what was then a beautiful abundant, and gentle place on earth.

My experience with Adam was wonderful. It helped me to face and accept fearful problems and their outcomes. I felt deeply connected with myself, others, and Nature.

I Learned to Know Myself as a Whole

27 year-old female, graduate student §

I had a guided Adam experience. Adam is an empathenogenic drug that my guide (a licensed psychotherapist) calls a "Gnostic catalyst," because it catalyzes a knowing which is already in the self, not in the drug. The Adam experience is one of expanded consciousness in a state of no fear, with deep compassion for self and others. Set in a therapeutic and spiritual context, a great deal of insight is possible.

It was for me a classic transpersonal experience: a profound and prolonged direct experience of myself and of the universe as a seamless whole. It marked a spiritual emergence of "Psychological Renewal though Activation of the Central Archetype" in John Weir Perry's terms, with elements of Shamanism and karmic patterns. In terms of Ralph Metzner's *Ten Classical Metaphors of Self-Transformation*, the major themes were Separation to Oneness, and Fragmentation to Wholeness.

I experienced dualism in many of its various forms: Mom/Dad, Male/Female, Left Brain/Right Brain, Good Mother/Bad Mother, Devouring Mouth/Loving Mouth, God/Goddess, Death/Birth, Self/Other, Subject/Object, Twoness/Oneness.

I kept coming back to the same answer: it's not either-or, <u>both</u> are true: polarities collapse once again into the seamless whole.

I went through a series of birth cycles, and I experienced myself as part of the evolutionary chain, as well as caught on the wheel of samsara, life and death. In the post-Adam experience, I was able to reconnect with fear, an emotion I've been out of contact with most of my life, particularly in relation to the medical profession. This enabled me to begin to remember authentic feelings I had forgotten, and to reassociate them with facts and memories I <u>had</u> retained.

---

§ *Set*: self-exploration, therapeutic.
Setting: friend's home, with therapist/guide.
Catalyst: 100 mg MDMA plus 50 mg MDMA.

Most profound of all, in terms of awakening intuition, was experiencing another way of knowing myself and the world, from the inside out, by being: knowingness from beingness. I learned to know myself as a whole by experiencing myself as whole, e.g., being whole. The hole at the center or core of myself became whole!

The days following the drug experience were equally profound. It's as though having once experienced my wholeness, all the channels had opened up, as though I had suddenly grown a vast, living nervous system. Insights and memories poured through me, fragments and pieces of the puzzle all started to come together.

In this altered state, consciousness radiated through and illuminated my whole being. I saw that normal consciousness is focused, like a laser beam which I can move about, touching only one small detailed part after another. Like a searchlight in the night sky, I have to keep it moving about, with "evenly hovering attention" to get an idea of the whole picture. Adam switched my laser beam to slowing, radiant light, and I also became the light—subject and object simultaneously, experiencing all parts of myself not separately connected, but as one. Inevitably, with such an experience, one begins to sound like a mystic, speaking in metaphor, feeling the frustration of describing such an experience from the limited, dualistic, language-making brain.

The Inner Warrior/Healer archetypes emerged kinesthetically in me as Tigress/Lioness. The Tigress with her stripes doesn't forget her past, is ever ready to savagely, if necessary, to defend herself and her cubs with tooth and claw. She also hunts and kills skillfully and swiftly, feeding and sustaining life. The Lioness, color of dried savannah grasses, lies in the warm sunshine after a meal and gently, lovingly, and tenderly licks herself and her babies, also nourishing body and soul. The same mouth, the same me, can defend and love.

Many more specifics of my Adam experience had to do with doctors and priests, and my attempt to bring them together into a true healing profession. It is possible to understand past life experiences in terms of the injuries and dangers I felt when doctors (healers) and ministers (spiritual leaders) function as intellects cut off from their hearts and bodies. My attempts to bring my body/mind/heart together in a spiritual whole has led me inevitably to the transpersonal perspective.

Finally, I brought from my Adam experience a willingness to really see myself, now that I had a larger perspective, and I knew that what I saw would have a different meaning. In fact, from that perspective, it was no longer a question of being critical or compassionate with myself. The question just never arose. What is simply is what is. I accept myself.

And I learned that in one way or another so much of what I have been struggling so long to attain already exists. One example is my desire and efforts to get my parents together. The fact is, two little packets of their essences did get together once, male and female, and I am the result. They are together in me. I am the embodiment of their wholeness. Like Morgaine at the end of her long struggles in the *Mists of Avalon*, when I contemplate the Whole, the Divine, I am struck with deep humility: "And I thought I could meddle in this?"

An after-effect of the Adam experience was the resolution of a problem with the state DMV. They had taken my driver's license away based on what I believed was an erroneous diagnosis of "psychomotor seizure." The drama that unfolded taught me the importance of the transpersonal perspective in medicine.I had always thought my so-called deja-vu experiences were a psychic phenomenon, in psychiatric terms, some kind of dissociation or hysterical conversion. My therapist gave me important psychiatric contacts (expert witnesses) who could corroborate my view, and psychopathology class gave me the terms to articulate it as well as the final diagnosis: Somatization Disorder, which features, among other things, pseudo-seizures. This diagnosis also provided yet another validation: a cohesive picture of my whole psycho-medical history from puberty onward.

During this experience I had to confront, in a heightened state of fear and vulnerability, various psychiatrists and neurologists (all strangers to me) in what felt like an initiation of sorts: trial by fire. I passed the test, however, and I was able to maintain my center in spite of considerably, heightened stakes and a lot of fear.

I emerged whole, with my soul intact. I passed the test and was pronounced "neurologically sound." I put together a strong legal case for myself (my lawyer said I really didn't need him) and I won. I got back my driver's license!

Born Again out of the Mother Star

37 year-old female, artist §

The journey began with "Ode to Joy," and my whole being seemed to flow into perfect peace. Soon I was listening to the tape, and began the journey back to my mother's womb, to my grandmother's womb, to my great-grandmother's womb. Time lost its meaning. Faces from the family of man appeared and disappeared. A new wave of light moved in and faces of men were living among the beasts: there were dolphins and fish and tigers and penguins and every living creature, and they were all born from the same womb. We were living in the garden of Eden, and life was green and lush and warm and simple.

I asked to see the first day of creation, and there was nothing to see. I was moving into something like a black hole, and life took on meaning in another dimension. I was far away, and felt a wave of alienation and fear. My mind made an attempt to take back control, but I knew it and was able to let go. The fear went away, and I was traveling back through the black hole. I seemed to experience death, and it was remarkably peaceful. The beings on the other side of death were radiating perfect love.

I walked through the door of my block and found myself in another garden. I moved so quickly, past faces and places and things. This part of the journey seems foggy. I remember faces and so many people. The people were all struggling for love and salvation, and many of them were in pain. I felt my body and their bodies hanging from the cross. The light fell upon us, and we moved into perfect love.

Their bodies began to move up in a circle and they were all saved. Then new faces would appear, and it would begin again. It seemed as if God held me away from them so I could see the cycle.

I saw all the faces in pain being touched by the hand of God, and the pain was transformed into perfect love. M stood up from her rock

---

§ *Set*: therapeutic, self-exploration.
Setting: at home, with therapist/guide.
Catalyst: 150 mg MDMA.

and began to walk around. Her compassion poured over me, and I recognized myself, and the "stuff" of the universes became perfect love. M began to tell me stories but I didn't quite understand them. Then I was sprinkled with dust and light, and began to wake up.

Later, same day: I was born again out of the Mother Star, and everywhere there was light. An Angel appeared in the company of doves and a Pegasus, and they guided me through all the universes. We traveled through a host of paradises: there were great clouds and an array of energies. Our trip followed the great light of love. We went through vast tunnels, and seemed to explode into new universes. They carried me into my mother's womb, and I began to take residence in my body. The womb was filled with holy water, and it absorbed some of my memory. I still knew the angels and doves, but couldn't recognize my being. The light of love was shining through the "stuff" of all the universes.

I am preparing to express my life on earth. I am home again and reunited with creation. And with all of this I feel there is so much more to be revealed.

Second session, one month later: the journey fell through my being as quietly as a gentle sunrise. At first it was delightful to melt into and travel through a blue, blue sky, and then oceans and forests and black skies. In a sudden, gentle flash my being surged with power, and I was resting in a lotus blossom. The blossom was drifting in a lovely pool of water. A gentle wind began to carry the entire scene into a circle, and soon "we" were whirling into light. The patterns of the light spoke to me, and I was filled with a language of no words. Another quiet flash and another wave of energy so intense that all the stuff of the universe became one magnificent light of love... and it fell through every level of awareness. This was the miracle of faith.

The energy lifted my eyes into the room and moved my body into a sitting position. The power of love was waking to every level of life. The confidence of love poured through every cell of my body, mind, and heart. My mouth began to speak though my heart: words weren't necessary, so I began to follow the commands of the language without words. A divine voice was giving me directions, and I was one with it. The energy slowly lessened, and I became like a child.

My Leaving Became My Homecoming

25 year-old female, student §

When I took the medication I took it as a cue to give myself permission to be totally for myself, and that any expression of love would be for me and it would be totally appropriate.

After ingesting the drug I wrote in a notebook: "I embark upon this journey, this odyssey unto me. Behold the love of God. Oh how I wish to go Home, Father. Take me Home. Love me. Take care of me this day and forever. Today is a day of learning, of gaining that which is termed wisdom, a becoming and a discarding of that which is the source of unhappiness, of all that stands in the way of me knowing my God-Self, my Christ. Behold unto me, Father, that which I be—God I am."

I waited. I didn't know what to wait for. I had asked for an unknown God to show up. Actually I think I just forgot to wait for something because all at once I found myself in a state of complete enjoyment.

As I lay, I felt relaxed and allowed for. There wasn't anything or anyone else to consider. As I was thinking of "leaving," I thought of all of the others present, including my brother, just as one might when one thinks about leaving friends. A deep feeling of immense love and gratitude welled, as images of passionately holding my brother colored my mind's eye. I knew at once to get up—not because I thought about it, but because that was my greatest delight, to be standing, and walking, and seeing the others. And I found my brother.

He welcomed my company and I was grateful for that. I held his head in my hands and kissed him and he was so sweet and I told him so. Everything was exactly as it should be. My leaving became my Home-coming. I thought I was going somewhere but I just showed up where I was.

I wasn't alone. I was being totally entertained, wholly consumed in the experience of Being. I was happening to myself. I didn't do

---

§ *Set*: spiritual exploration.
Setting: home, with small group and guide.
Catalyst: 200 mg MDMA.

anything. I felt, I listened, I asked. Not in an ordinary sense, though. Feeling, listening, asking were all the same, the same action, the same event. It was all Being, for every moment was absolutely immediate and there was NO TIME to do one thing and then the next. There was NO TIME to do anything, it was already being done. In every moment I was listened to, and spoken to, and I was told the answers.

I wasn't alone. We played and laughed. My breathing, had a soft, smooth quality that was offered no resistance by my body. I was actually breathing into my body. The breath went from without to within, but without a vehicle to do so. Imagine blowing up a balloon— without ever having taken a breath to do so. I became as enamored with my body as a child is with a colorful balloon. All of a sudden I had a body because I had chosen one, and in the choosing of it I was given it, and I was happy for that. I was surprised to hear soft, gurgling, laughing sounds, and my eyes widened when I noticed my hands were those of a small child.

At some point I became concerned about whether the others were being cared for and I asked about them, and I laughed in utter delight with the recognition of how my thought had limited me to terms defined by time and space. Here I was enjoying the direct presence of God and all at once I was worried that the others were left out. It dawned on me, or I was told, that the others were enjoying themselves in Gods presence, and there was no possibility that anyone had ever been or could be left out. I heard myself giggling again with relief at the obviousness of it all—the way it is.

So I let the world sit on itself, to lay where it lay. I put it down as though I had been holding it up, keeping it in place. I was free to roam and to move about, this tremendous burden having been relieved of me. Not only was I free, but this very action allowed for the absolute freedom of the others.

I remember feeling constricted at the thought of the experience being simply a drug-induced phenomenon. I rolled over on to my side, adopting a fetal position, as though trying to turn my back upon the Presence, pouting for fear of eventual abandonment. And then I was told, "You see, you have free will. I will never leave you—but you will." I smiled in recognition, relief, and gratitude. "When you are afraid, it is because you have stepped out of the moment. Love without fear is as simple as opening the hand." I watched as my hand repeatedly opened and closed. "Live it. Live it." And I told him that I would.

What can I tell you of my life now? I can make two observations regarding my life as a result of this experience. One is that I am not the same. I am more. I allow more. I express more of my love. I listen more. I am happy more. I play more. I laugh more. I feel more. I sleep more. The other observation is that I am the same person I have always been. I am more the same than ever.

I Surrendered to the Death of, My Outworn Fears

50 year-old female, therapist §

Before, my life was full of fear and doubt. Even though I had worked on myself for such a long time I had only been able to intellectualize (for myself) that we are all God. I could help clients feel that or touch it and I could heal them of assorted problems. But I could not love myself as I could love them, nor could I let much love in—as much as I wanted to. I began to work in therapy and I started to embrace my feelings, and in so doing I learned to accept myself.

I saw that I had to achieve an end to struggle, fear, and doubt in order to be free to experience love. When I was offered the sacrament I knew that I would take it, but fear and doubt and my alter ego had to be overcome sufficiently to conquer my resistance.

The experience was exquisite and remarkable. As I took the sacrament I experienced a never-going-back feeling. My higher self swallowed deeply. I surrendered to the death of my outworn fears and doubts. They were replaced with an incredible flow of joy throughout my body. I felt far away at first, and soon I was everywhere or anywhere. I was formless yet really alive for the first time (in this life, anyway). My higher self spoke to me and showed me many past lives as well as current life circumstances. I was lovingly forgiven for all the sins I felt I had committed.

At first I had a sense that I had arrived on a plane composed of the notes of the music, then on a plane composed totally of color. Everything was intensely alive and joyful. I found it so wonderful to be out of my body. I felt myself as my higher self, forgiving all of my lives and making them whole, finished, no more an influence now. I also felt that my migraine headache would now pass away at last, perhaps not suddenly, yet surely.

My body danced and leaped with the kundalini energy. I just let it dance, and I loved it. I knew that I could love and be loved. I felt

---

§ *Set*: therapeutic, spiritual.
Setting: home, with therapist/guide.
Catalyst: 150 mg MDMA.

that both were one. I felt safe, safe and secure. Occasionally the alter ego would make a comment that nothing had happened here that was important, and that I wasn't doing anything right! I was amazed that it was still trying to take me over. I simply lay there, loving myself, even with those thoughts. The thoughts eventually disappeared, and I asked my higher self to take me deeper, to show me more.

I feel I experienced death and its beauty, and I felt the dissolving of large amounts of fear. The first time I opened my eyes I felt my higher self looking out of them, with joy, love, and tenderness for all life.

My dream life has been exceedingly real, and I have been able to recreate the feeling of leaving and of returning to my body. It is an ecstatic and an unbelievably free feeling. I have experienced three very powerful dreams: one past life, one present but alternative life, and an experience with my mother (who died last November). My ability to be in the dream yet objective to it is even better than before. I feel that I can better understand prayer and how to pray. This is again a revelation, and I feel real gratitude for this privilege given to me.

I am trusting myself more in all matters, and I am more patient and forgiving. Yet I feel free to chose with whom to spend time. My intuition with clients is better. I am looking again at the Kabbalah, particularly the middle pillar, the Kabbalistic cross. I am finding creative ways to solve my financial bind. In fact I feel that it _is_ solved, and that, again, I am arriving at the place where the solutions are offered! I am looking forward to taking the sacrament again. It is a marvellous gift for communicating with my higher self. I feel so much closer to myself now. I believe that I will eventually be able to create this state and to maintain it when I so choose. I marvel at what lies beyond it!

My Body Dissolved Into Tiny Cells

44 year-old female, with breast cancer §

During the experience there was a continuous undulating or wavelike movement of all things around me or within me—such a soft, rhythmic flow in all things—constant feelings of bliss. I was the external fibers of a flower waving in the gentle flow. It was as though my body dissolved into tiny cells that were part of everything. There was a knowing that I must let go, let go, to allow the flow to continue, that any holding or trying to control would prevent the fluidity of life, would stagnate life.

I gave so much love and forgiveness to those who were around me that I became love—I didn't know there was so much in me.

I kept repeating "Just let go, just, let go" and as I let go I could feel the cells in my body moving towards healing. I became aware of placing my hands on various parts of my body in need of healing. The healing as occurring physically—I was the healing and I witnessed the healing. I didn't want to end this beautiful state, but I remembered my promise.

Afterwards, I was amazed at my own possibility—that there even existed such a bliss. I kept closing my eyes to return to the state.

The following morning, I realized that the very sore throat and painful shoulder had improved tremendously; they continued to get better in the following days.

For several days everything was so soft and gentle. There were moments of feeling the wavelike movements again, especially in breathing and experiencing Nature. I was looking through new eyes, knowing the most incredible fullness was possible. As the days passed, the memory didn't fade, but things seemed flat in comparison. I want that blissful state to be in me always. I am so honored to have had that experience, and to know the choices and possibilities there are for me.

(Editor's note: her doctor reported an overall major improvement in her health since her Adam experience.)

---

§ *Set*: therapeutic.
Setting: at home, with therapist/guide.
Catalyst: 150 mg MDMA.

I Saw Myself from the Creator's Eyes

36 year-old female, professional, invalid §

The Adam experience was a rebirthing, the guide was the midwife. Several predicaments in my present life had moved me to seek therapy: my relationship with a black man, my demanding and time-consuming job, disappearing friendships, the fact that my family didn't seem to want to know me, a tumor that might require removal of my womb, and a weirdly irregular heartbeat.

Most of my life has been an enigma to me. I have never accepted my family as being related to me—I never let my family be mine. I've rebelled, been wild, felt guilty, and punished myself, mostly with poor relationships. My friends find me surprising and complicated. I have always wondered what was wrong with me—why didn't I fit?

The Adam experience provided answers to every question I asked. I began to see myself, to hold myself as a mother holds a baby, noticing both my love for her and how beautiful she is. I saw myself from the creator's eyes: beautiful, loving, striving, growing, and often bewildered. I listened to me. I listened to my Self talk to myself. I had been disconnected so long from my inner voice. Now I heard comfort, praise, and love. I was amused with my confusion, but I was tender and forgiving towards myself. I got encouragement and advice. Clearly, unmistakenly, permanently I felt: I AM GOOD.

The answers and advice were marvelous. As I brought up each incident that bothered me, the undisclosed aspects of those enigmatic incidents turned out to be things I had forgotten about: what I had done that provoked them, the ways I had behaved, and the thoughts and decisions I had made which cut me off from the people I loved. I watched my part in why my life unfolded the way it did. Things had unfolded as natural consequences of my choices in each situation. I forgave myself and others for our natural responses to the situations we found ourselves in.

Next, I wanted to know what I could do about it all now. I saw

---

§ *Set*: therapeutic.
Setting: at home, with therapist/guide.
Catalyst: 150 mg MDMA.

scenes of me speaking what my heart has to say, and making peace with my Mom, Dad, sister, brother, boss, co-workers, and each of my friends.

I saw how truly I love my partner. I asked how my parents could accept him and be glad for me. I saw what to do and what to say. I saw our wedding in the home where we live together now, and I heard what my wedding vows would be.

All my failures were results of me trying to express my love. Failing doesn't mean that I am bad, or not good enough; it doesn't mean something is wrong with me, or that I should be punished.

For instance, I have been terrified of bearing children. I realized I was afraid God would punish me by giving me a deformed child for the "unforgivable" things I have done. It dawned on me that even if I did have a deformed child, it would be because that child would need the depth of love I am able to give, not because I should be punished.

I even was shown that my body could shrink the fibroid tumor I have. I saw my cells linking arms, as men carrying comrades off a battlefield, carrying out the cells of the tumor. The tumor has been shrinking!

The Adam experience is love. Knowing love. Experiencing love. I flow from the very source of love! A perfection in "things as they are." was revealed. I began appreciating myself, my circumstances, and the people in my life. Confusion dissolved. I felt at peace. Things seemed to fall naturally into priorities proper to the value of life. Life owned a fulfilling quality. I felt blessed. In a state of Grace. Pure and sinless.

I learned that indeed, I am a healer, a gift to this troubled universe.

Such enormously powerful lessons and answers. Such remarkable re-visions of myself. I didn't want to forget anything—could I lose touch with this insight? I was given four "signs" to remember by:

When I hold my left hand in my right hand, palms up, I will remember my precious heart, to be easy on it. I will remember the preciousness of all humans, to be easy on them, and to share love. I do this often when I am with people, particularly if anyone is upset.

When I cup a hand over an ear, I remember to listen to my Self.

This is helpful when I am confused, or distressed.

I cross my hands over my chest to remind my heart to beat one beat. It gives me courage when I am hesitant.

I bring my palms together in praying mode to remember to be humble, to accept what is needed and let go of my stubborn willfulness. It helps me remember that it will work out better to flow with the way things are, with God's plans.

There is a last result I am pleased with. I have always been too serious, and wished I could laugh. I chuckled quite a bit during the experience. Now I laugh more easily and more often at myself and at life's funny situations.

Adam is a gift, a blessing, a "sacred medicine," as my guide referred to it. It is soft. It is truth. It is love. It is grace. Adam had a wholly positive influence on how I live and how I feel about life.

Seeing into the Beauty of One's Being

35 year-old female, businesswoman §

Sunday morning: not quite 24 hours since my encounter with Adam. A new day is beginning. I feel soft. I feel present. And I am filled with my spirituality.

In many ways yesterday was a spiritual experience. I am moved by my love and by my connection with God. I think for quite some time I've been somewhat out of touch with that I remember one morning not too long ago, as I was putting on my nylons and heels and my silk business suit, my "armor," as I refer to my work presentation, I said "I feel like I'm losing myself." Adam was an opportunity for a return to self.

It was also a completion of the past in some ways. I am moved by how clearly I saw my mother's death, and how peaceful I am with that. I am very aware of my mother's connection with God, and of her gift of love and appreciation. I'm committed to carrying that forth, and expressing it in the world. And I felt compassion and forgiveness for my father. I am really appreciating who I am in all of this, my experience of love and how all right everything is with me.

I remember when the power of Adam was at its peak, I felt that I would be carried away, that I would go unconscious. The guide told me to lie down, and I wouldn't. Maybe I didn't surrender? I felt like I was holding on. And I gripped the pillow, and the sofa. What would have happened if I let go? I had intense body sensations at the peak. I felt like my brain was going to explode through the top of my head. My jaw chattered and clamped, and I chewed the inside of my mouth and the sides of my tongue with my clenching teeth. I felt for sure I was going to throw up. I remember perspiring. My face and hands were wet.

The intense part seemed quite brief. There was a fast and steep climb from the beginning to the climax and then a rather gentle and long denouement with the end coming around ten in the evening,

---

§ *Set*: therapeutic, self-exploration.
Setting: at home, with therapist/guide.
Catalyst: 200 mg MDMA.

when I went to sleep. I took the tryptophane, but I did not sleep well.

I'm more aware than ever that I have a particular model of the world. Suffering is something I'm grappling with. Yesterday I saw that my view of the world is just that, a view. Yesterday created an opening for me, an opportunity for me to shift my map of the world. Yesterday was also a completion around my experience of being a woman. This male female thing has been an issue in my life. There's something I saw that allowed me to appreciate being a woman in a way I never had before. Again, there's an opening, and it has to do with being fully powerful, and being a woman. I also experienced compassion for men. I remember saying "God made men, too, so they must be OK."

I go back to work tomorrow after being off for two weeks. I feel apprehensive. This opening of the heart is lovely. As I said before, I feel soft. I have the thought that this is too vulnerable a position to be in, that I seem to need to harden up, to get my armor on, in order to go out and function in the business world.

I want to stay "opened," full of heart and love. This is where the joy is, and the possibility of life as celebration. As e.e. cummings says, "Since feeling is first, he who pays any attention to the syntax of things will never wholly kiss you...."

Monday evening: I got through Monday. I felt quite emotional most of the day. I suspect it has something to do with having had an experience of Heart, of being in touch with that which we're really all about, something of essence, of spirit, of source, of our deep sensitivities, our humanity, as contrasted sharply with that which most of us interact with on a day-to-day basis: concerns about making money, treating each other shallowly, dealing with numerous seemingly unimportant details, playing political games, driving in rush hour traffic, not "connecting." What I need to do is to be in whatever environment, whatever circumstances, full of heart, and love, and spirituality. To bring peace and joy to whatever situation. To have a light heart, an open heart.

Tuesday evening: I had a great day. Nothing particularly special happened in terms of circumstances. I realize that when I have a "bad" day, or things are not going right, I wonder to myself "What's wrong with me?" And when I have a good day, I take it for granted, as if that's the way it's supposed to be. Today I decided to take credit for having a "good!" day. Today, three days after Adam, I would say that what stands out for me is the potential Adam has as an aid in breaking up one's reality, and for seeing into the beauty of one's Being. I want to underline the importance of the context—created for the experience. It would not be the same experience without a wise and loving guide.

Thursday evening: I've had a fantastic past few days. I'm really loving this new appreciation of being a woman. Something actually happened for me: I am done with trying to prove something. There's still some unsorted stuff in this area, but I do think I've shifted things. There's something I know about being a woman that I didn't know before. And this impacts on one of my goals: to appreciate myself and express myself more fully.

Brand New to This Planet

39 year-old female, psychologist, ex-alcoholic §

Approximately fifteen minutes after taking the Adam, my head began to feel out of kilter and my body more relaxed. I began to feel vulnerable and childlike, needing reassurance from my sitters that they would not exclude me, or ignore me. As people talked, there was a "zing" to their words as they first spoke.

I continued to regress, becoming a very young child—a creature who seemed brand new to this planet, a very innocent being full of curiosity and vulnerability. There were wonderful energy releases in my body, especially in my jaws, where I carry much tension. I found myself continuing the sounds and the facial contortions I had made during the breathing.

At first I needed nurturing, and I needed reassurance from those around me that they accepted my strangeness. My sister encouraged me to look for acceptance from within, and that helped me to get more within mysell At one point I sucked the breasts of one of my sitters. It was wonderful and fulfilling to nurse from her as we sat on the rocks in the sun by the ocean.

Throughout this process my mind functioned at different levels: the "judge" was judging that it was inappropriate for a grown woman to nurse, and was I a latent lesbian; the therapist part was going "Yea! You're having a Good Breast Experience!" At the same time I was an infant, surrendering to the sucking process.

Having received from those around me, I was now ready to be alone, and to go more within. I had a sense of being guided by my inner and outer teachers. I was taken back through my life, and given fuller explanations of the various turning points in my life. I uncovered deeper understandings of why I am in certain relationships, why I have felt and acted the way I have, and why others have acted as they have. It was very valuable to me at this time, as I had been going through a period in which I was experiencing much self-doubt, guilt and regret

---

§ *Set*: therapeutic, self-exploratory.
Setting: home, with friends/sitters.
Catalyst: 150 mg MDMA.

regarding the decisions I'd made in this life and regarding my behavior in many relationships. There was clarification of the various tests and training I had been receiving in this lifetime and of the direction in which that was moving me.

It was also brought home to me my areas of vulnerability. I saw my misuse of mind-altering substances in this life, and in past lives my resistance to letting go of the high. It was mandatory that I be willing to dance with the whole process, and not cling or push away any part of it. Also, I saw that in the past I'd had shamanistic powers, and I'd misused them. I went on ego and power trips that resulted in my involvement with the dark forces. At this point in my life it is possible for me to open to my deeper powers again as long as I remember that I use them in the service of God, and not for my ego.

The whole experience. felt like an initiation. It was frightening and exhilarating. I was urged to be more physical to be more in my body, which contains the secrets of who I am, the blueprint for my unfoldment.

The intensity of the experience decreased, I felt a profound sense of deprivation and a desire to be back where I was the moment before. Then I would gently tell myself not to cling (which is what I used to do when I drank) but to let go and experience the present moment. The anxiety dissipated and there was a sense of peace and contentment with the new level. The key over and over was to not cling nor to push anything away—just as the Buddha taught.

Upon awakening the next day I felt anxiety in having let go of so much control the previous day (though I never felt out of control), and I felt sad that my boundaries made me feel so closed up again. For the next few days I moved in and out of being able to open and to let go more, then bringing in my old boundaries. I now understand more clearly how I close myself up.

I look forward to returning home and exploring my relationships with various family members using the new information I received. I am grateful that I now know underexperientially that there is so much more to me, and to life, than I perceive on a daily basis.

And Love to Season the Soul

28 year-old female, professional model §

On the Adam I had an experience of loving myself completely. There was no question but that I loved myself and that love was the backdrop of life.

The next day I wrote: My love, I am with you as you play. I Am you. I love you. Be tender today. Let your heart open to the love I show to you. You are the most precious prize here. You are that which the universe turns for. Awake. Breathe. Live in abundance. Together we live our dreams. Now that you have discovered the I that was already here, I may play with you, as one. Live freely. I shall take us to the stars. There will be no us. Do not forget me. These love poems are the entrance to forever. I will come to you again soon.

And someday soon we shall go to other universes, and see and understand greatly. Learn as much as you can here. Open up as much as you can, and always love change. I have loved you through your tears. I have loved you through the hatred. I have loved you through the passion and insecurity.

Beingness is JOY. This age of beauty shall bring a change of attitude. No longer outside beauty but the inner heart, the beauty of the soul. Unlimited beings. Acceptance. Joy. Adventure. All shall come to hear of the awakening Christus…the joy within each of us, that we shall soar again and again.

Never mind what they think. They may call you weird and crazy. Yet they see the Joy. They are drawn to your light. Breathe and let the light in, into them and to you. You need only love them, for I shall work wonders. We shall go and bring light into the planet.

I see aura lights. Unlimited vision. Joy—opening up to the experience of Joy. I will send great money straightaway, and love to season the soul. We long for the experience of opening up and becoming one with one another. The heart opens so that there is no thing between the two bodies now. The experience of Joy shall be

---

§ *Set*: self-exploratory, spiritual.
Setting: at home, with friend/guide.
Catalyst: 150 mg MDMA.

ours, an upward, spiral growth, an ever unfolding feeling and emotion. Though I speak of you/I/we/ours, we are one. The awakening Christus has the remembrance of all that is inside.

Yet no longer shall we be separated, you and I. I am here for you always. I shall take you from this plane when we are done. Yes, we can come back, of course, yet we shall be together. It is a very great lesson that you have learned, to allow me through you, to allow me into your life. We are returned together as One, to grow faster now into that which you want to be.

The following day:

I now feel and know that I am the eyes, ears, feelings of the spirit. I feel so safe, so protected. The Holy Spirit is myself. There is no mystery anymore. We are here to do, to feel exuberant. My soul has taken me through all of the growth emotions, to bring me back to the lovely place where I am now. And the holiness is me. I am holy, for the grandeur to which my soul aspires now is Joy.

We are here to experience, to do what our thoughts are, to manifest. I now have safety, security, when I am scared: I turn to my soul. I AM. Still, I used to be afraid of that. My soul is split from a soul that we will merge with again, my soul mate. That is there. That is not as important to me—yet—as finding my own self. Yes, that soul mate is myself, too. I revel in the insight into feelings, in sadness, in joy. The breast opens and movement stirs in my heart. I breathe through my heart. The center of gravity has shifted in my body.

I turn to my soul. I long to hear its sweet voice again, to speak as my soul, to move consciously as my soul, my self. After making love with my lover, my Self told me that we would learn how to enjoy pleasurable love and that I should open up so that I could teach myself. I spoke of love to myself, to be able, loving, far different from what I had experienced before. The words were about how I would learn that people loved me; and I him, and much love through love the song of Govinda, Hare Rama, played for me. I went into love, back to myself. Words of pleasure.

Baby Floating Through the Universe

43 year-old female, housewife, mother of two §

A heavy weight is coming down, flattening me, pushing me down. A big weight. Then a cool breeze. I'm pushing my way through a wind tunnel, an enormous force is pushing against me. After I make my way through it, I'm in a light, open space. It's as though I've gone from one room to another. No part of me is enclosed, encapsulated. I had to push against the wind that was pushing against me in order to get into the next room. I feel all of the different parts of my body. Sometimes I feel just the very tip of my nose, like a little block of wood. My legs feel really heavy. I don't feel anything under my hands (which are across my belly). I just feel them. Sometimes my body is just gone.

A cool breeze comes now and then. My lower arms feel deep, I can feel the insides of my bones. It feels wonderful. I'm surprised that my mind is still here. I don't feel anything scary. It all seems familiar, like home. I'm home. I'm going home. It's deep, floaty. I'm going. Wonderful. I feel my bones. I might throw up, my stomach is not upset but there is a little knot. I might throw up this knot that I am holding. Everything is nice, feels wonderful, I'm going. I'm surprised that my mind still works.

An awareness of being here, beyond here. Both. The setting is important. Very deep, very far, galaxies, very far out there. Spacious, open, dark. Some visual patterns, thin lines of bright colors, rapidly changing. Mostly floating, like a baby through the universe. That's what it feels like. Floating through existence. Infinite, the whole universe. All that space and me. Never ending, floating through it. I'm home, finally I'm home. My legs are more trembly now. I'm sweaty and I want to stretch out.

I didn't think about myself. It was beyond ego, beyond my personality. I couldn't believe that the experience lasted four hours. Questions about where I was seemed not to apply. It was great. Thank

§ *Set*: self-exploratory, spiritual.
Setting: at home, with friend/sitter.
Catalyst: 150 mg MDMA plus 50 mg MDMA.

you. Real gratitude, I was always wanting to thank you. I felt so grateful. I loved the feeling of the wind tunnel. The best image I have is of a baby floating through the universe. I felt like liquid, like water. I felt like home. I remember what Augustine said. Something about the heart always being restless until it finds its rest in God. I felt that complete rest, no searching, finally home.

Deep, far-away galaxies, a spacious, open, dark, floating existence in the infinite, whole universe. Wonderful.

Individual Experiences—Men

Peace with Great Energy, Tangible, Expansive

53 year-old male, minister §

On the morning of August 18, in the presence of two others, who also took MDMA, I drank 120 mg of MDMA. Prior to taking the substance I was handed a rose, freshly cut, and I was made to feel loved, safe, and secure. Even so I was a bit anxious, because, except for a single encounter with a psilocybin mushroom, I had never ingested a psychedelic.

After a few minutes I began to feel numb from my head to my toes. I became frightened and I looked to the rose for re-assurance. The numbness gave way to a sensation of great energy. It felt as though every molecule and atom of my body had a powerful motor, and for the first time every one was turned on. The great surge of power and energy was overwhelming and I began to have second thoughts about taking the substance, but I knew that it was too late. I was at the highest peak of the roller coaster, about to descend with the speed of a falling rock. Great excitement and fear held me, and once again I looked at the rose and felt re-assured.

All of this had the feeling of me versus it, and it was winning and was very much in control. Then, at some point, the struggle and fear vanished and a great feeling of peace came over me. It was not the kind that comes from not having problems or stress, but peace with great energy, super peace, tangible, expansive, a real thing, and highly prized. I sat until I was sure this state would not dissolve. I felt as though I were breathing for the first time in my life.

All the while I had been looking at the desert sand beneath my feet. Occasionally I would raise my eyes and look at the pile of wood stacked neatly beside the garage. If the wood appeared so fascinating and wondrous, what must the mountains, which were at my back, be like? I thought perhaps if I turned to look at them, that I would surely

§ *Set*: spiritual exploration.
Setting: outdoors, desert/mountain, with two friends.
Catalyst: 120 mg MDMA.

be overcome by their great beauty. So I turned very slowly, each glance being a bit longer, taking in more of them with every turn of my head until I felt confident enough to stand and have a panoramic view of the whole range. They were spectacular and <u>breath-taking</u>—literally. I was filled with joy.

I went over to my fellow travelers, with much excitement, and I exclaimed, "I knew that there must be such places as this, I knew it, I knew it." Part of this realization was from having read about such states of consciousness, but the larger part of it was that I felt at home, like the birds or fish who migrate thousands of miles because somehow they know and are called by an inner prompting to a place where they have never been, have never seen, but at last find.

Then came a flood of connections. I felt connected with some master plan. Everything seemed to have a purpose and a plan, a reason why, and I felt caught up in it and was thrilled. Life seemed to have been conspiring to get me here to this moment, to this place of love, beauty, goodness, and truth. There was no uncertainty about any of this. "Only the fool, fixed in his folly, thinks that he turns the wheel on which he turns." The greatest freedom is to have no freedom but to go where we long to be. I had been migrating for fifty-three years in order to be home at last. I knew that I had done something as great as the birds and the fish.

As the heart quickens the closer you approach your destiny, so I saw the connection between the fact that my body had uncontrollably quivered the day I had interviewed as a possible candidate for this experience, and the greatness of the experience to which I felt called and which was now part of me. I felt as though all that I was trying to accomplish in life was somehow confirmed by the experience that I was undergoing. It was a premonition, and a confirmation. I was being caught up in the mystery, and the providence, and I was able to know the feeling and the certainty of it all.

I looked at my friend and I knew that he must be an emissary for a new way of living. The feeling was one of destiny. I was enjoying my destiny for the first time. It was real and I was realizing it.

I wanted to explore, to walk out into the desert to stand alone in that vast panorama of beauty. A few hundred yards from the house I found a huge stone, about five feet high, into which the wind had carved a seat. I climbed onto the rock ("ta es petros"—you are the rock) and sat there in the hot morning sun, looking up into the blue sky, breathing wonderfully clean, warm air, surrounded by overpowering mountains, great rock formations, and ancient boulders that, I had been told, were 25 million years old. I knew what consciousness was about. I thought of the destiny of mankind. We were going to the stars.

I walked back to the house filled with awe and wonder. I asked whether we could go swimming in the spring-filled pond, which was down a gentle slope, a few acres from the house. We nestled there amid three and four-story high rocks and boulders of great beauty. Here in this idyllic setting of monoliths and cattails, desert and lush vegetation, I decided that I wanted to be baptized, without ceremony, ritual, or words.

Coming out of the cool spring water I felt refreshed—cleansed inside and out, totally alive and especially privileged.

The rest of the day was spent hiking and mountain climbing, eating rich, hot soup and being fully into the here and now. The intensity of the morning had drifted into a pleasant transition of fun, closeness to one another, and to the events as they unfolded.

Sitting at night under the stars and distant lightning I knew that I had come into an awareness as unique as life and into the promise of scripture, "I have come that you may have life—and have it more abundantly."

Adam Reveals Emotional Truth

37 year-old male, psychiatrist §

My wife and I took Adam together, to deepen our relationship and communication. There was a great closeness, trust and joyfulness between us. I felt elated, and I was confident that I could better all of my relationships with everyone I knew and cared for. I said to my wife, "You know, I think I could give my mother an Adam session now."

My relationship with my mother is not an easy one and she would of course not approve of drugs. As soon as I said it I felt sick and threw up. I was surprised and chastened, although I still felt very accepting of whatever occurred. Then my wife pitched in encouragingly, "No, I'm sure you could do it, and I'll help and support you on the trip." Whereupon <u>she</u> threw up, and we both laughed uproariously.

Adam, we realized then, doesn't necessarily promote bonding between those who are estranged. Rather, it reveals <u>emotional truth</u>, what's true for you now, both the good and the bad, in regard to your feelings towards others.

---

§ *Set*: self-exploration, relationship communication.
Setting: at home, with partner.
Catalyst: 100 mg MDMA plus 50 mg MDMA.

MDMA Experiences Have Saved My Relationship

37 year-old male, businessman §

What is the experience like? I address this by describing what my partner and I do. Mainly we sit on the floor facing each other and gazing into each others' eyes MDMA is the eye contact drug. Physical contact is also maintained, so we have eye contact, hand-holding, gentle caressing of hair and face. Skin surfaces and hair feel incredibly soft (a feeling that persists well beyond the four hours). One is impressed with the preternatural beauty of one's partner. No one has ever been so fine, delicate, exquisite, or full; the sense is that she is all and everything. "I have been looking all my life for you."

I believe that the love experience on MDMA is the Divine Love spoken of by the saints. There is suddenly an openness to giving and receiving unconditional care and adoration, one feels privileged and blessed, nor do one's ordinary fears and defenses rise to quelch these powerful positive feelings. Without question the experience is powerfully intense—powerful, but unlike the overwhelming experiences on LSD or mescaline.

This intense love for one's partner leads naturally and immediately into sexual areas. I desire to undress myself and to have my partner similarly unclothed. I enjoy touching my own genitals and having them touched, and I enjoy touching my partner's. But all of this seems to be an aspect of a greater love, and the genital contact has a charge that is little different in character and degree from an exchange of glances or a facial caress. The world, too, is observed as clear and profoundly present—here and now, in Gestalt parlance. A color slide of a wall whose paint is peeling appears stunningly beautiful, as though seen for the first time.

One night my partner and I held each other while we watched the full moon rise over the ocean and reflect on the waves. We

§ *Set*: enhancing communication, relationship.
Setting: at home, with partner.
Catalyst: 150 mg MDMA.

experienced closeness while we experienced the wonder of the world. In my experience, sexual consummation—that is, orgasm—is impossible until the end or slightly after the MDMA experience. If a distinction can be made between love and sex, MDMA is a love drug, and not a sex drug. This fact, taken along with its raw power suggests that one would not want this experience with everyone, and one would not want it every day. Experiences of this significance require time to digest, so intervals of two weeks or more between experiences seem appropriate, the positive nature of the experiences notwithstanding. As this is a drug that feels sacred, one does not want to profane it by mundane usage.

Further comments are called for on the interactive qualities of MDMA, particularly on the verbal level. Conversation emerges spontaneously and comfortably from the contact and closeness. My partner and I were able to express total love for each other, and the level of articulation is reminiscent of classical love poetry: "A loaf of bread, a jug of wine, and thou...." The accumulated grievances of a stormy five-year relationship paled into insignificance. We didn't forget them, indeed we talked freely about them. Yet the unpleasant memories, the laundry list of hurts, had no charge; it was just data, like yesterday's weather. And most touching of all are the expressions of gratitude for the gift of this beautiful life and for each other. It is this receptivity and appreciativeness that Catholic mystics call Grace.

A handful of MDMA experiences have saved my relationship. My partner and I had actually broken up, in each others' and in the world's eyes (an announcement had been made). We had been falling apart despite our love for each other, a rich family life, and an adored infant child. Under the MDMA we reconnected with our mutual caring and love, with what was important to us, and with the place of our love in the larger religious and spiritual nature of things. The lessons we learned carried well past the drug session. We have a look that we give each other that instantly takes us back to the caring place. The MDMA experiences are centerpieces of our common mythology, they are shared peak experiences. Sex is better than before.

Examining My Emotions with a Sharp Lucidity

32 year-old male, writer §

My statement of the session falls at a turning point in my life and career. I want to examine this transition and let myself proceed as quickly as possible to the task at hand.

My greatest hope is to have a long life, to spend my spirit, to find somehow, through love, the communion of my soul. This is shrouded in mystery, feminine, a sacred marriage, something that is spoken of in all of the sacred realms. It may take me a number of years, and I hope that I have the strength and the joy to carry forward; and as an old man, perhaps, to look back and cast even greater joy onto the waters. The joy of the sage, the one who has worn himself away gradually, is not like the street fighter, not like a drunk, not like a damaged man (referring to Dylan Thomas). He is like one who has worked hard for his wisdom and knows that he can last...that he can last as long as he wants to last. That's very moving. That's very human.

The strongest beneficial qualities of MDMA for me were the following: 1) Enhanced presence of mind. 2) Stimulation of speech without loss of articulation. 3) No strong side effects to confuse or to distract cognition, logic or continuity of thought. I certainly surprised myself, but all to the good. MDMA was discursive, labor intensive, and it examined with a sharp lucidity my emotions, and organized through memory and speech my many thoughts and perceptions, arranging them into a pattern.

I gained important insight into the history and development of my personality and character. Awareness, confidence, and self-assurance improved. The session provided me one of the best opportunities I have ever had for true self-examination. I felt refreshed, vigorous, alert, and happy to an unusual degree.

---

§ *Set*: transition point in life.
Setting: at home, two therapists/guides.
Catalyst: 125 mg MDMA plus 50 mg MDMA.

As a result of my session, my hopes and expectations were fulfilled, but it would also be fair to say that following the session I experienced a mild form of emotional inflation.

I discovered and understood with a positive and profound conviction that my identity and personality were intact. I had feared, I suppose, that I might find that I had been damaged in some irreversible way. I felt tremendous relief and joy when I learned otherwise.

Regarding other people I had a feeling of great loyalty. I realized that others, many others, had helped me along life's way. This feeling touched me very deeply. Regarding the world itself, I felt glad more than ever to be alive in this world, and I felt joyful, even euphoric.

Honoring Our Differences

42 year-old male, college professor §

I took 2CB alone, in order to explore my relationship, which had been marked by many arguments and bitter disagreements over the past year. During the session I talked with my partner in my mind, from the heart. I understood that one of our patterns was creating more and more separation between us.

She would mention a difference in our attitudes that disturbed her, for example that I was promiscuous. I would respond by saying that I was "inclusive." Then, in our usual way of relating I would try to minimize, or smooth over, our differences in order to avoid an argument. I would argue that I could be monogamous if she wanted me to, that I had been so before, even with her, etc. All of this would only lead to another argument.

During the session I suddenly realized with emphatic conviction that I no longer needed nor wanted to play out that pattern. I no longer wanted to minimize or smooth over our differences. Instead I made a new commitment to myself. Since I loved her just the way she was I would accept the differences between us, indeed I would honor them, respect them, and even celebrate them. The French phrase, "Vive la difference!" came to mind. I saw that in honoring our differences we could begin to search for common ground and build the relationship on those expansive areas of commonality. It is no longer necessary for the other to change in order for me to be myself.

---

§ *Set*: self-expolration, relationship focus.
Setting: at home, alone.
Catalyst: 25 mg 2CB.

Meditation and Remembering the MDMA State

32 year-old male §

I've waited a week to put my thoughts and feelings down on paper; I am just now coming out of the euphoria of the experience. This past week I have been happy, contented, loving, concerned, easy to get along with, and at peace with myself. I've made a concerted effort (and it hasn't been that hard) to retain the self I was put in touch with.

Regarding the experience itself, I had no awareness of the passing of time. Throughout I was comfortable personally and I was completely at ease with everyone present. The physical sensation was a combination of warm heaviness and mental clarity. I was totally involved in the conversation and interaction with my friends. All inhibitions and defenses were stripped away, so that I was directly in touch with my feelings and my ability to express them. My thoughts flowed with reason and purpose. I felt a genuine warmth and affection for my friends and a strong desire to express my love and concern for them. I was able to say the words I've saved for so long for fear of prying or of hurting them.

The greatest reward was the positive feedback I received, the respect for who I am and what I have done, and this has given me a far greater feeling of self-worth. Seeing myself through others' eyes has enabled me to see more clearly the good that I have to offer, and it is now easy for me to throw off the cynicism I've been hiding behind. I want to build on a new foundation of trust and openness and to accentuate the positive forces within me. I would hate for it to sound like the gushings of a Pollyanna or of a recent convert to the latest cult. I honestly feel that I was given a rare opportunity to look inside myself and to gain a profound understanding of who I really am.

I feel that through self-revelation and the comments of my friends

§ *Set*: therapeutic.
Setting: at home, with therapist/guide and two friends/participants.
Catalyst: 100 mg MDMA plus 50 mg MDMA.

I gained a greater awareness of my strengths as an individual The session brought out my positive aspects and these overshadowed a negative self-image. It was a profound, delightful experience that I continue to benefit from.

The experience has stimulated my interest in self-discovery. I now feel that I have a great deal of potential that is untapped. I have begun reading books of a spiritual and philosophical nature to help develop this potential. I have resumed meditation after a lapse of about six years; it has a calming, centering effect that helps me remember the MDMA state. I hope to continue meditation on a daily basis and to go farther into it than I have in the past. MDMA has helped me to find my center while meditating.

I have taken steps to increase my self-awareness, and I have re-evaluated my needs for love. I think my self-confidence has increased due to the improvement in self-esteem.

Now I Feel the Pain as an Ally, not as an Enemy

45 year-old male, writer, arthritis sufferer §

During the past few years I have been afflicted with a very painful case of spinal arthritis. Until recently there had not been a day when the pain was not present in most parts of my body. At times it has been so debilitating that I could barely move for days at a time. I have tried a number of prescribed drugs, including Motrin, but none has had the noticeable, long-term effect of easing the pain and the attendant worry, concern, and even depression.

Until recently, in February, 1984, I began to use MDMA, with the idea of easing the constricting arthritic pain. With only a minute or so of my ingesting the substance there was a noticeable decrease in the pain. As the day progressed, I felt my body become less and less constricted. For some months I had hardly been able to walk more than a few feet at a time. Now my body began to move freely; doubts and fears connected with the disease dissipated. I felt a new sense of hope as the "arthritic crystals" appeared to be breaking up, releasing the very tight constriction. For several days the pain, while not altogether gone, was greatly alleviated. For the first time, I had real hope that, with the aid of MDMA, I could reverse the patten of living in constant pain.

Other sessions followed, with similar results. At times my body felt so free and light that I began to dance and move quickly with a suppleness that I had not known for years. On June 9, I ingested the substance and, again, within a minute, I began feeling elated, and the spinal arthritis pain that had been great before was alleviated.

On June 23 there was another session. Seven minutes after the initial dosage the pain in my back began to disappear. Then I began to focus in on a healing spot for my arthritis—a point at the lower back that, when pressed, relieved pressure. The muscle constrictions

---

§ *Set*: therapeutic, to heal arthritis.
Setting: at home and outdoors, with partner.
Catalyst: 100 mg MDMA plus 50 mg MDMA plus 50 mg MDMA; series
 of sessions

became less and less, and I felt I was really beginning to be in touch with my body, which was in a state of fluid motion. I felt that there was a healing effect surrounding my body. Then I went into a frenzy of movement and I felt the heaviness and constriction leave the body. The hard stiffness in the lower back and knees loosened up.

During this experience time stood still as I looked at the Taos Mountain with a sense of Oneness, stillness, quiet. The stillness of the mountains and the mesa became absolute, the only reality, as a consuming inner heat began to burn. I began to focus on a healing spot for my arthritis, an acupressure point at the lower right back, lower chakra. After applying thumb pressure there, I began to expand and I felt love energy from the mountain enter my heart chakra.

I felt a strong connection with space and the planets. I was part of them. My origins lay there. I played Gustav Holst's "The Planets." The music of Mars coursed through me. I was in space again, the Void. I was at home, free. Mars, the bringer of war. I saw conflagration, the history of the world in battle, but it was a cleansing. From the conflagration came a period of understanding, wisdom, and love. Pockets of deep understanding amidst the fire and conflagration.

I felt a tremendous closeness to my friend, and a great warmth. Space surrounded me. Both my friend and I were still there. We were part of space without time. I felt us billions of years in the past and billions of years in the future. We were part of the universe. A great love permeated me. My friend was a large part of it, but so are the world, universe, and beyond.

I focused in on myself and felt like a different person; consumed by warmth, with a wonderful feeling. My body was in a state of fluid motion; muscle constrictions dwindled, and I was in touch with my body.

Touching the earth and reaching for the sky had a healing effect on my arthritis. Warm, free, beautiful. Dancing, free-flowing body movements, a frenzy of movement, then quiet. I felt the body freeing up. I was literally blowing heaviness and constriction from my body. Energy was caught in my throat. The body was really free. There was a sensual feeling about it. The hard stiffness in my back began to loosen up. Energy was running up my spine, loosening the stiffness in the spinal column. I was literally bouncing to the music.

I felt the presence of space beings all around me. They were trying to impart some message, but I was not open enough yet to receive it. I felt that we all have a benevolent tide of extraterrestrial beings surrounding and protecting us. They want us to grow, to expand.

My body felt like it was opening up to something, like a clear channel. Energy attacked the jaw. I felt the beings trying to get through my body. Still no message, though. I felt the night sky, covered with stars. I felt a real closeness to the <u>aliveness</u> of space. The arthritic pain returned; I felt a slight headache as I came down.

An additional session followed one week later. Within ten minutes of ingesting the drug, there was a considerable lessening of the back pain. Later I again went into a frenzy of movement as insights began to appear as to how to begin to control the energy flow within my body. There was a very rapid movement of my hands, and the arthritic constriction in the hands, knees, and back loosened considerably. My body moved very freely, and I felt much better. For the first time I really believed that I could be cured. Somehow I felt I was beginning to integrate a new me, free of pain. The arthritis in the knees and legs disappeared, and the back pain rapidly decreased.

During this experience I moved with awareness into my body. I felt that my body was a temple that I had desecrated. I wanted to let the body go, but I realized that I couldn't. It was telling me that it would continue to rebel. I felt as though the body were ready to explode in all directions. It felt heavy. I was very much in a "the-body-is-not-me" mode. I felt powerful eruptions from the inside. I felt I needed to go through a death experience—symbolically, I hoped, but great fear was there.

Then I felt comfort, a joyous knowing that there was no death. The body became much freer, though the arthritis pain was still there. I began a frenzy of actual, physical self-flagellation: a very rapid movement of hands, a loosening of arthritis in my hands, my knees, and my back. I lost consciousness while going through fast movements. My hands shook and I could not write. I shook violently and began to exhale rapidly; I was close to hyperventilation. My body moved exceedingly freely, my legs in particular. My body really freed up. I could tell that there was still some arthritis there.

Ferocious anger set in, and my hands started trembling again. My legs shook frantically again, particularly my knees, where the arthritis pain is centered. I breathed heavily, and I felt very, very hot. I felt that I was burning up. A feeling of death surrounded me, but a certain uneasiness and fear prevented me from experiencing it. Still, somehow I knew that there was nothing to fear.

I suppose what frightened me was the feeling that I didn't want or need the body any longer. Yet I was stuck with it. Still, I was not my body. I felt an unexpected confusion, but the fear subsided. I began to feel the eternalness of things, unseen things, the real things. A roar was bearing down on me, like a freight train. I felt that I wanted to do something drastic, but I was not sure what. Consuming fire burned me, I felt that my body could burn away. I thought of spontaneous combustion.

There was something present that I had to break through. I felt that this could be the key to loosening completely the arthritic "crystals." I almost lost consciousness in another frenzy of movement and self-flagellation. I beat my breastplate. The energy had loosened considerably, and I felt much better physically. I still felt some remnants of the arthritis and it pissed me off. I was going to beat the son-of-a-bitch if I had to flagellate myself to death. Beating myself seemed to help, and now I was beating myself with a regular broom. Energy had left the breast/heart area and travelled to the back. My friend beat my back and shoulders with the broom This brought a big improvement, and my energy freed up.

For the first time I really believed that I could be cured. I felt anger at myself and at my body, and I beat myself with a whisk broom. I felt as though I were caught in the middle of a battle, and I was determined to win. I was fighting the bastard and this felt good. The fire was burning me up, consuming me. I felt exhausted, I was coming down. There was much improvement in the body, but each little pain made me angrier at not being able to let go completely.

My body then shook fiercely, and my exhalations became heavy. I lay on the floor and frantically flailed my hands. I grasped the flesh around my midsection and pulled hard. I beat my butt against the floor, hard, shouting as it hit. Energy travelled up the body to the throat. I grasped my throat and shoulder as though I wanted to rend the flesh from my body.

I felt very hot again, and I feel great anger at myself. Damn it! I wanted to flail the body, beat it into submission if necessary. Then there was quiet. I began to feel a love of myself, for myself, course through my body. It was very, very freeing. Some pain was still there, but I was determined to get it. The pain returned to my back, and I sat in it and just felt the pain. Tears came to my eyes. There was a feeling of sadness, and perhaps of loss. Somehow I had to face it and find out what it was. I was fearful because, perhaps for the first time, I saw that I was destroying my body. Somehow that had to be overcome, for otherwise I was in danger. Perhaps that is what the earlier closeness to death was tying to tell me.

The clouds were so still and quiet. I felt a powerful oneness with space; I wanted to leave my body and join that oneness. Death felt closer and closer, and I felt resigned to it, but I drew back. I had to discover what this thing was in me that wished to die. I knew only that my body was not important, but that I couldn't drop it yet. What was this death inside me. Where was the Life? Perhaps both were the same. I felt that there was a connection, a kinship between them. I felt I must experience death, symbolically, but I was afraid that it might turn into a "real" death.

I began to try to feel the death experience. I felt great sadness at first, then body movement. Surprisingly the fear left and, briefly, I passed beyond the portals of life. An encompassing, beautiful white light radiating love surrounded me and, for the first time, I knew that death was not to be feared. It was not the end-all. It was a beautiful, new beginning, a rebirthing. My friend gently massaged my back, pushing the energy up into my spinal column.

The pain is not all gone, but for the first time I know that it will be. I feel a renewed sense of life and purpose. I realize now that I had got to such a point where I was either going to let the negativity and pain kill me or else I was going to rid myself of it. I feel strongly that I have chosen the latter, though more work still needs to be done.

Oh, God, the glory of feeling, the love. For the first time I feel the pain as an ally and not as an enemy. I can use it for insight and understanding, and not for self-destruction. I no longer feel the pall, the aura, of death around me. The pain is telling me that it will disappear completely only after I have pushed that invisible "integration" button. Why? The answer comes as tears flow, and the heart, as it expands, seems to <u>know</u>. <u>Using</u> the pain with love and understanding instead of constantly fighting it with deep animosity will enable me to end it. A "bolt" from my heart caresses my pain and, strangely, I feel a deep love <u>for</u> the pain. It is my teacher. By accepting rather than rejecting it, wonderful, soothing clarity about it pours into me.

On July 18, I had an experience very similar to MDMA, without taking the substance. My feelings and actions were very much the same, however. The energy began to move through my body and I began to move—stretching, pulling, shoving, guiding the energy somehow. It did not blast through the arthritic blocks but appeared to dart around, over and under them. I felt great relief. Later in the day I began to breathe in the cool, wet, soothing wind. It had a comforting, even healing, effect on the arthritis. I exposed both my front and my back to the wind, and the effect on the pain and constriction was noticeably good, and healing. For five full days I was almost completely free of the arthritic pain—the longest stretch of pain-free time in three years!

On July 23, I had stiff another MDMA-like experience without ingesting the substance. Once again my body moved at a rapid pace and the constriction loosened. I seemed almost to push the constriction down and out of the body through the gut area, which became loose and free. Then I began physically to pull the arthritic pain from the lower back It worked. The energy went to other areas of the body.

Wake Up! Wake Up! Before It's Too Late

26 year-old male, graduate student §

It was my third MDMA journey session over an eight month period and I was really up for a journey through my personal universe. The session had been well-planned with a written agenda of personal issues, cosmic music, and an agreement with the guide to keep the experience internalized as much as possible with eye shades, earphones, and minimum conversation.

While listening to the *Neuronium* album by Chromium Echoes, I was caught totally by surprise and was thrust into a state of outrage by the mind-jarring sound of an atomic explosion. In that expansive and highly amplified state, I felt like I had just lived through an atomic bomb. It was real, very real, and I felt like my reactions were in the space between the blast and the last few milliseconds of my existence. All that was missing was the physical experience of the thermal wave and vaporization. The rest of the experience was extraordinarily real!

The experience thrust me into a state of total disgust, anger, and rage—rage against those who persist with this madness in the face of the evidence. And I felt outraged with the most extraordinary human rights violation of all time—an outrageous violation of the right to life for all living things and the feeling of helplessness as we teeter at the brink of extinction.

Intensely passionate, and trembling with emotion, I expressed my disgust, anger, and rage, which were recorded by the guide and are transcribed here word for word from the tape of that session: "That's unbelievable, unbelievable! That's so pathetic and so sick! That's what one piece of sound brings up for me. There are people all over this planet who are running around saying, Wake up! Wake Up! Wake Up! Before it's too late. Wake up! Before it's too late…

---

§ *Set*: self-exploratory.
Setting: at home, with friend/guide.
Catalyst: 100 mg MDMA plus 50mg MDMA.

Wake up! Before it's too late.... Wake up! Wake up! The potentials mankind has—and destroys!!!!!"

(Editor's Note: one year after this experience, S finished school and began to devote himself full-time to disarmament work.)

A Sense of Passive Urgency

69 year-old male, professor, author, activist §

The following are verbatim recordings from the session:

I'm wriggling out of a snake skin, and I think I'd better stay with it....

In the beginning I focused on the bringing forth of my first consciousness other than ordinary... was centrally... the recognition and commitment that has to do with a <u>deep</u> spiritual center....

The question you asked about the universe we're in, the view we hold... around finding a part of the... all over oneness... certain things stand out....

It's like having a quiet conversation with the unconscious. There's a band of light behind, inside and outside, to fit things around, an experience of different aspects of perceiving.

It feels as though the central thing is to see what this other kind of consciousness is, what it is trying to say through me. I passed the state where what comes to be remembered... as though part of my mind I recognize as dealing with this question: Who answers these questions? <u>That's</u> what wants to be talked about.

What we're trying to do is respond to various things in the picture. The original intention I came in with was to learn anything I could to help me, to create this planet, to say "yes" to deep intuitions...

Suddenly, with a look of Aha!:

My goodness, who decides what experience comes forth? It's a tussle, a fight between two different parts of myself. There's a sense of passive urgency: it makes a difference what we do, but getting frantic won't help.

A feeling as to the immediate meaning: a speed-up in personal life, correlation with the speed-up in the planet. I sense a more active

---

§ *Set*: exploratory, planetary consciousness.
Setting: at home, with two friends/guides.
Catalyst: 100 mg MDMA plus 50 mg MDMA.

role. My life will be more centered, less distraction.

Something will be different... even more serious than before.

A Spirit Moved through All My Meridians

45 year-old male, therapist §

As I rested and waited with my eyes closed, I meditated on the prayer "I am infinite love." I knew that I was safe. I knew that wherever this journey would lead, wherever might happen, I was safe.

As the spirit of the sacrament moved, I felt enveloped by love. I felt very certain that all that there was in the past, is now, and always would be love. I am surrounded by love. There was a strong sense of choosing. I could choose to create the illusion of fear and pain, and live in that, or, have the love. I recognized having spent enough time living in the dark.

When I felt totally certain of my choice...there appeared a series of faces. It was as though I were viewing a slide show. They were all people I was compatible with; I hadn't trusted their intentions in our relationships. Now I had the clarity of knowing that I had never received any less than their total love. The confusion had been my fear and doubt. In the instant that their faces appeared, our relationship healed. The outstanding aspect was the instantaneous awareness and healing.

A long series of vibrations followed. It was as though a spirit moved through all of the meridians, first superficially, then deeper, to release all blocks or barriers. At first it felt like a gentle massage, or rocking. At times the intensity increased, a sense of laser-energy moving through the deepest parts of my being.

The higher energy felt like a purification, a sense of being blessed, bathed after a rite of passage. The end feeling was a physical sensation of rebirth...the child of God made known, released from years of accumulated encumbrances. At points there was a feeling of weight lifting off of my body. The armoring, the protection accumulated over my lifetime, lifted, and the opening was bathed in light.

---

§ *Set*: self-exploration, healing.
Setting: at home, with guide.
Catalyst: 200 mg MDMA.

There were visions with many of the releases. I witnessed the choosing of sickness as a way of declaring boundaries, a sense of self—creating pain to avoid pain. I was able to watch myself as a child, interpreting the world and creating a way of dealing with it. With other releases there were feelings rather than visions. Opening up the pelvis released many old messages about sexuality, vulnerability, and protection.

At times there were rooms with doors that opened. One room held what appeared to be a pile of ashes. When the thin layers of ashes were blown away, the room became a bed of crystals. The crystals spent most of the time locked in the room, buried under the ashes. Another room was full of tissue (epidermis), which was tender, with many irruptions and lesions. Spending a moment focusing tenderness, the tissue healed and became baby soft and smooth.

When the vibration and flowing of light diminished, there was a sense of quiet, of small chattering in the mind. I chose to move away from the chatter to see whether there was something that I was avoiding. Was this ego? Was I avoiding darkness, a fear? I floated into a fold, with a sense of moving, flowing inward, softly being swallowed. Quiet. Moving farther in.

I was happy to see my friend. We went home. He commented that I seemed more available than he had ever experienced me. We rested and went to sleep early. I woke frequently during the night. I slept physically and psychically closer to him than before. I had many dreams, many messages, and a few "aftershocks" (spontaneous vibrations).

I've never felt so flexible. My body moved so freely. I felt like an infant who hadn't learned limitations of range of movement or body—a wonderful feeling. No aches. No tenderness. My body felt open.

My overall sense of the passage was that of an opening, the most incredible move inward. I sense that there is more inward movement to be made—both with the sacrament and by focusing on the everyday plane.

Desire Transcended by Being Fulfilled

48 year-old male, writer §

I did an experiment, at a California health and spiritual retreat center, comparing massage with and without Adam. The first massage session was "straight." It was beautiful—by the sea, with warm breezes wafting in; and the masseuse was naked and beautiful. Lying on my front, with my head turned towards the side, I opened one eye and saw a perfectly formed breast outlined against the shimmering blue sky. I fantasized and wished that we were making love, caressing instead of massaging.

The second experience was with 100 mg Adam, and the masseuse also took 50 mg. The massage seemed longer and slower, and my body responses were much deeper and more total. I felt blissful. I recalled my wanting and desiring her, from the first session, and I realized that I did not have the craving or desire now; instead I felt as if we were making love! The desire was transcended by being fulfilled. I no longer wanted anything else than what I was receiving, which itself was perfect,

I understood that this was the essence of <u>tantra</u>: transcend the pull and the fascination of sensual pleasure and desire, not by denying or punishing it, but by fully accepting the experience as it unfolds. This is it!

---

§ *Set*: self-exploration, healing.
Setting: outdoors, in massage center.
Catalyst: 100 mg MDMA.

In the Womb, When the Light Was Primary

22 year-old male, college student §

I want to recount my experience while on Adam. As I lay on the mat after first taking the drug, I became greedily upset that the drug didn't seem to be working. I was so hungry for the drug. Just before my guide asked about how I was feeling, I felt the first rush of sensation.

As the effect became stronger I was surprised to feel pain. I had expected euphoria, and I felt that I was doing something wrong. When the guide asked again how I was doing, and I told him that I felt so much pain, he told me to go into that pain; that response freed me to have my experience and to go deeper. My breathing became shallow and spasmodic.

I think what came next was feeling myself beginning to spiral upwards from my body. As I spiralled up I broke through memory into my infancy. I was so sad and alone. I was a baby that couldn't find a mommy to comfort it when it was in fear. I was a baby coming out of the womb on the first day of it's life, looking and seeing no one to greet it, as the most special nascent and fragile beautiful being. The baby's heart felt so pressed by coming back into the world without a face to look at the baby with awe and wonderment. That baby hurt so much. Where was that baby's mommy?

The baby looked backward in time. I'm looking for a time before the sadness, for a center that doesn't reek of the sadness. I'm floating in the womb. I still hurt. The womb is filled with my mommy's pain, but at the same time I don't know the difference between me and mommy, and mommy's pain is my pain. I know now that the heart is a light, but the light is so gripped by the pain that I can't rejoice yet. No, perhaps I don't want to rejoice. I hold onto the pain, but I don't know this during the Adam or during the baby time. The baby

---

§ *Set*: therapeutic.
Setting: at home, with therapist/guide.
Catalyst: 150 mg MDMA plus 50 mg MDMA.

in the womb is looking for a time when the light was primary, to a time before the pain to serve as a foundation for the baby's life.

I knew that my mommy hurt. The day after Adam I took a hot tub and was in my mommy's womb again. This time I looked at the sun that was the heart and I saw the light, and I saw the clouds of pain around her heart. Maybe I was going backward to find a cure for my mommy. The baby knew about joy, but didn't know how to give it to mommy. Baby felt so much compassion. The baby is a sperm from daddy. Daddy is contaminated. He hates his penis place and the poor sperm babies that live there. Daddy doesn't give my sperm baby to mommy as a wonderful gift. He saddles her with me. The sperm baby has the bunched, ugly face of hate.

After going back to the sperm and still not finding a place before the pain in my life, I come back to being the baby. I see the light as a radiant fire. The sadness is still there but the possibility of light is brighter at every moment. So many babies come into the world, all with the possibility of being such radiant creatures. The poor babies: they need to be taken care of.

My First Sense of Not Being Paranoid

33 year-old male, graduate student §

I went into the experience seeking greater empathy for the child I once was and still am, and to know my own emotional needs well enough that I could begin clearly to distinguish my needs from those of others. I intended to explore the feelings I had in early childhood, particularly in reference to being abandoned by my mother at five, in order finally to begin to rid myself of the burden of this depression.

I also wanted to explore the issue of work and financial survival, of how I could work at a job—to earn money—without falling prey to that kind of depression that comes from not having my needs met while serving the needs of others. This has always led to an exhaustion that I have found crippling and deeply discouraging. How am I to earn money and have my deeper emotional needs met?

The issues of emotional differentiation from my mother and of financial solvency/independence are very closely related. The connection was and is a major issue for me to explore.

For the first twenty minutes or so of the experience I felt considerable fear. I felt myself lowering down into a softer and more vulnerable place. I could feel the layers of fear peeling off of my torso and moving away into space.

I felt immersed in fear for a time. Soon after ingesting the second capsule, I dropped below the fear and contacted a warm and supportive baseline feeling, a place of support that was totally without fear. This gave me my first sense of what it is like to not be a paranoid, to be like other people.

I did not return to childhood memories as I thought I would. Instead I remained in the present and experienced my issues in condensed form within the context of my current relationship. My issues of fear, financial survival, and emotional dependency all fell

§ *Set*: self-exploratory, therapeutic.
Setting: friend's home, with one other participant, two guides.
Catalyst: 150 mg MDMA plus 50 mg MDMA.

within the relationship. I felt very clear that I didn't want to return to childhood, that there was no need to do so. I didn't feel that I was resisting or avoiding anything; I needed and wanted instead to contact the heart and to establish an ongoing connection with it. This did happen.

When I listened to the tape of my experience I discovered that I have indeed been carrying out the intentions I had during the Adam experience. As long as I remain in contact with the heart and am open and honest with my relationship partner, I know that my childhood pain will continue to surface and to resolve itself within a context of healthy mourning, and at a pace that the bodymind will decide is appropriate to my capacity. My partner understands and accepts this.

Being in the Center of a Sphere, Breathing

28 year-old male, poet, programmer §

I found the session extremely enjoyable. When it took hold I felt a glowing warmth in and around my heart, and my entire body felt as though it were full of moving, gelatinous warmth. Very pleasant.

The primary realization that I came to during the session was that most of my problem areas (depression, health, job) have to do with cutting off the flow of energy that is available to me on Adam. My feeling, with that energy moving through me, was that if I could allow that movement to occur, and allow, that movement to direct me (like the wind blowing a sail), my life would work itself out quite naturally and without too many problems. A large concern of mine has been what other people might think of me—and with that energy moving in me I found that it didn't matter what other people thought.

One image that stayed with me and which I felt often during the session was the feeling of a golden fountain flowing through my heart—almost an actual feeling.

Another image was that of being in the center of a sphere, breathing, and feeling myself in the center of hundreds of rays that formed a star with me in the center. Along with this was the feeling that if I could stay in the center of that sphere, as the center of the star, that I would be directed and moved in the correct dimensions.

I realized places where I stop myself from giving and receiving in relationships. I related the feeling I had during the session to an experience I had when I was an infant, and I was attended by a beautiful golden light while I was crawling in a bean patch. I was able to see that my mother loved me a great deal—and I contacted a memory of when she was holding me as an infant, something I had lost.

Afterwards, one of the most useful revelations from this session

§ *Set*: therapeutic, work on depression.
Setting: therapist's office.
Catalyst: 150 mg MDMA plus 50 mg MDMA.

(so far) has been that I notice that I do not run very much "Father" energy—and I characterize this as energy of authority, purpose, and assurance.

My second session with Adam was a solo—I took it without a guide. One of the issues that I wanted to work on was being more comfortable with being myself. I made arrangements with a friend to come four and a half hours into the session.

I went into an amazing vision, not really a vision, because it was more intense—it was more an experience. I felt as though I were in a chamber with walls of light and air in the shape of a pyramid. And everyone I had ever known (this life, past lives, future lives) was there. I felt all of them, some more than others (experienced as brighter lights amongst an assemblage of light beings). I felt overwhelmed with love. I felt the presence of my mother (dead for three years) and I talked with her about not loving each other in the past, so let's do it now. The two of us sent love to various other people, including the brother of a close friend, and my father.

As before, the journey was extremely pleasurable physically— warmth and movement of energy all through my body. As before, all of the issues that I brought to work on seemed very easily resolved. Many of the realizations I had centered around love.

In particular I realized that it is "right" for me and my partner to love one another. I realized that I want to bring this love experienced during Adam to my life. I realized that I can love people whether I'm with them or not.

One issue I worked on was being more joyful. I realized that all I have to do was to <u>be</u> more joyful—and it seemed crystal clear how to do that—simple <u>be</u> it. It was the same for vital energy—all I had to do was have it, to want it.

I worked extensively on blocks to creativity. They seemed to be centered in the area of my Hara (two times I asked to be shown where the block came from). I received three images, one of being a rock with a vein of something else in the area where my stomach (hara) is, one of being tortured in the inquisition in Southern France (this also had to do with something I had written), and the third was of something Egyptian.

At one point I took a shamanic journey into the underworld. I ended up in a large grove of oak trees. I buried four eight-sided crystals, one in each corner. I then stood in the center with my two helpers, a cat and an eagle, and I danced. There were many people dancing with me, leaping, with warrior energy, and I had a sense that my (male) guide was there dancing with me.

After that I walked on a trail with my animals until we came to a section of run-down warehouses where I had been before, both during lucid dreaming and during shamanic journeys. I went partly with the intention of finding what was there for me. I saw a little boy running. I realized that he was a part of me, and the space became brighter. I saw a little girl, and now she became a part of me. And then five different friends came up and became part of me, and the whole space was no longer a run-down warehouse but was full of light. I saw a little baby and I said, "Come here, little friend. Come here! I love you!" Then the little boy was in my heart.

I've noticed several differences in my behavior since the trip. I no longer feel fearful around people or intimidated. I feel much more sure of myself. In general I feel less in a hurry. I notice a growing resolve in me of wanting to share with others, and a resolve of wanting to be involved with people and to share my writing and music.

The Infinite Bliss of Being a Conscious Entity

30 year-old male, compulsive sexual masochist §

This session was different from the other one, right from the start. The first words on the tape are, "I feel tingly all over. I feel real happy, not speedy or excited like with acid, but just calm and happy to be here enjoying life."

The ultimate problem I see here is almost metaphysical. How does one describe perfection, bliss? At the same time the descent from that state was experienced as a falling out from perfection and bliss, of being pulled away from something very beautiful and true. This experience I have found to be intermittently painful and wistful during the past couple of days.

I didn't have a lot of specific recollections of suppressed material from the past. Even when I had what seemed to me were unmistakable birth-related experiences, I did not find a lot of mental accompaniment to what was happening to my body. My mind was calm, floating easily, relaxed, and was noticing what was going on with equanimity. It was strange and beautiful. There were none of the actual mental regression, the images and sounds of birth that I remember from LSD sessions. The body was just going through its thing and the mind was completely comfortable with that.

If so much beauty and calm is possible, I thought off and on, why do I have to suffer so much physical tension and unpleasantness? It was so bad at some points that I literally felt waves of despair rise up in me. As I watched, those waves would recede. And going to the hot tub in the evening returned me completely to the state of bliss I was in at the time of the drug effect. And yet the waves returned.

I found myself looking forward to the next opportunity to take Adam but I was somewhat ambivalent about that. I didn't really think that it was a matter of fearing that I could become addicted to the

---

§ *Set*: therapeutic, self-analytic.
Setting: at home, with guide.
Catalyst: 200 mg MDMA plus 50 mg MDMA.

experience in the sense of being addicted to alcohol or to sexual excess with prostitutes. I perceive those as addictions precisely because of their compulsive quality; they have such a compulsive quality because, by definition, they are characterized by the experience of <u>never actually obtaining a satisfying, whole, pleasant experience.</u>

With the experience of bliss that is available with MDMA, on the other hand, I feel none of that compulsion. I feel no desire to go out in the street and try to purchase MDMA for my own use. I don't find my thoughts turning to it constantly, as I have with the sexual addiction. It really has an entirely different quality, it's in some way outside all the time, outside of my life and my neuroses, literally a taste of the infinite bliss of being a conscious entity.

It is a rare and great privilege to have had this experience. In a very fundamental sense it is the kind of experience that every conscious being really wants and needs. We get a sense of our true selves and how they are perfect, beautiful, whole, and complete. It fulfilled all of my childhood dreams, all of the unfulfilled longings, and all of the feelings of loss and limitation have been swept away by the sense of who I really am.

What I'm really talking about here is what is, to me, the fundamental thing, the basic reality of all realities, and it is this: that my nature as a conscious being is that I am infinite, I am bliss itself, but at the same time I am in this finite body, both with shocking suddenness into this really strange world, burst forth from my mother to spend my time and then to return or move onto the timeless existence that I have always had.

In my feelings I experience the fact of birth as one of not wanting to be here. That is, I had that experience at birth and in feelings I have had it again. Now I am not thinking of checking out of here. I'm not crazy, but perhaps only too sane compared with my usual state. What I am tying to describe is a feeling, not an intention.

I remember saying in awe and wonder to my guide at one point that I found it so shocking, so unexpected, that I could experience my birth, that I could experience that taste of infinite bliss without going through all of the feelings of panic, fear of death, physical agony, longing for sado-masochistic destruction, etc., that I had convinced myself that I had to go through. I had it wired up that I had to pass through those gatekeepers before I could deserve or "qualify" for unity.

It's like what I have been trying to describe: it was almost too deep, almost so far outside of or deeper than my previous consciousness that I don't know what to make of it. I would just encourage everyone to do it—because what better gift to a conscious entity is there than to make available a taste of this bliss, this perception of one's true nature?

All during the next day I kept slipping into a really odd state of mind where the reality of our infinite existence as beings would suddenly come flooding in on me. Walking about the streets or driving in the car I kept thinking of how we take on bodies, sort of get together and make agreements to come to this planet and go through these experiences in bodies and look at all of the peculiar dualities we have set up here on this world.

In the Land of the Gods

30 year-old male, professional §

Before the experience I thought it might be a bit hallucinogenic, like mushrooms. I thought that I might trip on concepts and reality. I really didn't know what to expect; perhaps a very sensual experience in my body, like really experiencing sound, movement, or taste. Actually my basic level of attitude was one of boredom. After money, sex, and food, what else is there?

During the experience I discovered that I have choice at levels of existence not known consciously to me before. Land of the Gods— beautiful beings, truth and wisdom everywhere, existence in an ocean of love.

I struggled somewhat at first with some fears about letting go, but I surrendered to the energy. I saw glimpses of the past, and of future possibilities. I saw and understood the meaning of all those whom I love and who love me, at the level of soul the level of the naked truth of myself. I discovered that I could heal myself, that I could erase negative patterns from my soul, and create new ones. I saw my soul-mate in this incarnation and how deep is the love between us. I understood the meanings of the moments in my life. I am grateful!

I feel that I have changed greatly during the past few days since the session. I see things very clearly. I see the truth in myself— relationships with others, my level of service. I have been crying a lot out of gratitude. I am moved deeply by the simplest things. My emotional self and body have been going through changes. A rash on my hands and neck has surfaced, but I am calm and strong inside. I just observe and stay connected with the bliss. I feel that I have increased my responsibility in life—indeed I am a god.

My love for myself, for others, and for life keeps growing. I feel a deep patience that I never had before. It comes from a deep peace

---

§ *Set*: self-exploratory.
Setting: at home, with guide.
Catalyst: 200 mg MDMA.

in me. I have travelled to many places in the world, but during the past few days I have travelled into the farthest reaches of the universe, far beyond my wildest dreams. The past few days have been my greatest travel adventure so far. I watch my little egoic mechanisms arise and I dissolve them in a sea of love. Life—whatever its purpose and direction—let it come!

The Continuous Embrace of Shiva-Shakti

55 year-old male, teacher §

At the beginning of the Adam experience there was the usual dance, but the visuals were far less. Then deep breathing began. My experience of this was far deeper and more prolonged than before. Then I began something that might be called "toning"; it was a new experience. I would sing one low tone for what seemed an interminable time. I can remember feeling this vibration in my solar plexus and in my abdomen. I then sang another note which was higher, again for a very long time, and again part of my body resonated to this vibration. This time it was my solar plexus and heart.

Then the song began. At first it was similar to an American Indian chant, although it was more lyrical; then it became more like a mediaeval minstrel, or the song of a troubador; then it had the feeling of some Middle Eastern place. Finally the song became English and it was a love song to the Earth: both the planet and my body. Magma, fire, and earth were the elements emphasized, and they seem to be the most operative elements in me. Magma is the conjunction of the opposites fire and earth. When I think about this, I see the Sun and the Earth. It is as though fire represents spirit, as in the Holy Spirit, and tongues of fire. Incidentally, my favorite holy day, Pentecost Sunday, the descent of the Holy Spirit, was celebrated the following day.

After the song, the image of the key came up. There was a discussion of responsibility (ability to respond) and my feelings about my body. My sense of responsibility has been excessive and burdensome. The key is a key and a lock, which unlocks the separation of spirit and body, allowing God to come in through the whole body. It is also the symbol of Osiris, the djed pillar. At this point, after tracing the symbol of my body, I felt the heat coming up my back for the first time.

---

§ *Set*: therapeutic, meditative.
Setting: at home, with male and female guides/therapists.
Catalyst: 150 mg MDMA; 3 hours later, 100 mg ketamine.

Then the ketamine session began.

When the guide adjusted my hands so that my arms were perfectly crossed over my chest, I saw a golden green casket in the form of a sarcophagus. I realized that I have been trapped in that casket almost all of my life—in the sarcophagus of excessive responsibility and other programmings. In effect, in many ways, I have been dead. Also, I have given pieces of myself away, scattered like Osiris; and I have lost my phallus to the crocodiles, my shadow symbol. I have seen the body and sex especially as unpleasant, disturbing, an experience to be avoided. It is also as though I'm waiting for an Isis (Aphrodite, Ishtar, Astarte) to make a golden phallus for me, to help me transmute my ideas and experience of sex and of the body.

Then I became extremely hot and I saw my flesh melting away, leaving bare bones that also melted away (this sequence was in bright colors). It was then that I felt that I was cosmic orgasm. I was "nothing and everything." I was united with everything. The melting of the body seems to be the melting of old forms within the body, samskaras. After this, I felt free and released.

When I was dissolving I saw a huge vortex moving into itself like a wave breaking. The vortex covered my whole visual space. It was of pastel colors, pale blue, pink, and lavender, and it seemed to have a texture with it. At the same time I felt that I was the vortex. I was neither going into the vortex nor going out of it—I was turning into myself. This was a most sensuous experience. Yet sensuousness does not come close to describing this experience. What comes to mind is that this is the experience of pure consciousness and of energy merging. This was a creation, a cosmic orgasm.

The guide asked me, "Who are you?" My response, after a long pause and in a voice that I could not possibly recognize, was "I am the one and only." My associations to this are that the Monad is the ultimate god from which everything emanates. My feeling is that of an extraordinary primal being.

I seemed to continue to work with this. Next I said, "I am the King of the Dance." I again had a feeling for this but concepts and words were hard to find. The obvious relationship is the "healing dance" I do in these sessions. The healing dance is the result of the release of energies, the dissolving of energy blocks so that perhaps in some way I can heal through these energies.

Finally, I said, "This is the most egotistical statement: I am God." At some levels I know and accept that I am God, but the negative programming, ego, etc., always pop in to hinder this being completely actualized. Some part of me will not let myself become enlightened.

Immediately after I said that I was God, I had an image of three necklaces. All three formed circles, one raised above the other. I couldn't see what the topmost necklace was made of, because all that I could see was a brilliant, clear light. The second was made of brilliant rainbow lights, but the third was made of intricately and ornately designed purple stones. To me this seems to be a visualization of the three statements of "who are you?" The uppermost one of brilliant white or clear light is the "I am the one and only." The second brilliant rainbow seems to relate to "I am the King of the Dance" and the purple stones relate to "I am God, the Self."

I had an image of a giant and beautiful vagina in the sky. My previous image of the vagina was as a huge black hole that could suck me in. This relates to the "open womb," the fear of being sucked back into a state of undifferentiation, the mother complex, etc. The vagina in this session was beautiful, it was of luscious pink, orange, and red colors, It glistened and had pearly drops of moisture on it. Somehow I relate its shape to a heart and I relate it to the painting of Venus rising from the sea, standing upon an iridescent seashell. My head is drawn to it when I look at it and it is exciting. The idea of oral sex had always been revolting to me before, but not now.

I am fire and earth. My spirit is fire, inspirational, intuitional father fire. My body is earth, material, sensory, maternal earth. The two together are magma, explosive and powerfully moving, the center of earth existence and the center of my existence. It is my heart where the spirit and body meet. My heart is magma—the love energy that attracts and acts, the love energy that cannot be stopped, that reshapes the earth, that will not change from its course. It is a power that transforms.

Creation is a continuing cosmic orgasm. Creation does not mean coming from nothing, rather it is the continuous outpouring of the "One and Only." It is the expansion of the "one and only" into consciousness and energy. It is the continuous embrace of Shiva-Shakti, both as one and two. As one and as two it is ecstasy. This continuous cosmic embrace and ecstasy are continuously re-enacted, echoed between lovers and by one who loves himself. The realized one, or saint, is always in this cosmic embrace.

Love is not a burden. Love is lightness, joy. The experience that I have had of love is that it is heavy, it is difficult, it is painful, it has meant responsibility, it has meant taking care of someone. All of that has burned away and these things are not the essence of love. Love is a spontaneous outpouring and a spontaneous reception. It is delight, play. It is not entrapment, but freedom. It is the freeing of my Self.

The feeling of freedom (being out of the Osiris casket) and of being together (parts reassembled) continues. I now realize that I can do almost anything I want—I can freely respond to situations and circumstances. The constrictions I felt before are no longer around.

The greengold casket was transmuting, just as the training in "responsibility" has been preparing me for the ability to respond. The demands that have been made upon me, which in many cases I have blindly accepted, have developed in me the capacity to respond. Now this ability to respond is detached from the programming, and I am really free to use this ability.

During the ketamine session I had the experience of being a totally clear observer of what was happening. I also felt completely stable. The two together seemed to be an experience of enduring absolutely pure consciousness.

Group Experiences

Around Us Huge, Mythic Archetypes Stood

35 year-old male, writer §

The drug first became known to me as a shift of colors toward golden and rose tones. Pigments in the room became intensified. Shapes became rounder, more organic. A sensation of lightness and rivulets of warmth began sweeping through my body.

Bright lights began pulsing and flashing behind my closed lids. I began to perceive waves of energy flowing through all of us in unison. When I sighed with pleasure, others moaned in unison. I saw us all as a grid-work of electrical energy beings, nodes on a bright pulsating network of light. One of the other participants later reported the same visualization.

Then the interior landscape shifted into broad scenes. Dali-esque vistas were patterned with eyes of Horus, brocades of geometric designs began shifting and changing through radiant patterns of light. It was an artist's paradise—representing virtually the full pantheon of the history of art.

Up and around us huge, mythic archetypes stood. They were sphinx-like, tall, ominous, shadowed, sometimes like the Assyrian and Hittite winged lions, then shifting through archetypes of temple guardians from old religions and from those of planets that I had not seen before—ancient, alien cultures.

About an hour and a half into the trip I was seeing my visions with my eyes opened or closed; and I was travelling to other planets and dimensions. In each realm a religious ceremony was in progress. On one plane, there were huge, mantis-like beings that were wise, sepulchrally dignified, welcoming me with their ritual. On another plane, green, gold, blue, and purple beings that looked like small, crystalline insects shaped and re-shaped in kaleidoscopic formations,

---

§ *Set*: exploratory.
Setting: group of 17.
Catalyst: 150 mg MDMA; 4 hours later, 20 mg 2CB.

sending me urgent messages of mute import.

Finally, a dimension appeared where all was crystal life forms, all were incredibly beautiful energy beings, on both micro- and megascopic scales.

Many in the group were experiencing wild hallucinations, but the themes of crystalline beings, Egyptian forms, and light-beings seemed common to many of us on later comparison.

The energy waves were radiating through me from a central, circular channel located around my pelvis. My thighs were shaking. If I stood up, I could direct the energy through my spine, and out through my limbs. During all of this time all of us could converse with each other at will. When someone entered the room, we could decompress to an ordinary level of reality. We were not overpowered, but self-guided. The vibrations did not have the annoying buzz of some LSD, none of the potential nausea of mushrooms or cactus psychedelics, none of the overweening love of psilocybin, but had instead an appropriateness, a calming, centering, and powerful sense of peace. With me, it then slowly became apparent where the energy waves were coming from.

It was as though I were hovering, several layers of obfuscating reality above a great howling source of light. As levels of misconception, representation, illusion, consensuality diffused and dissipated like a clearing fog, the sound grew louder and louder. It was the sizzling of an arc-light of billions of volts, it was a roaring of a thousand suns, it was the sound of the universe ablaze. As it became more apparent, it was a huge, round ball that I was now orbiting. To call it white light would be to pale and daub this light monochromatic. It blazed with a radiance that was primordial, with an intensity that was absolute.

I came to know—not through language but through innate cognition—that this roaring explosion was life itself. It shrieked and pulsed through everything living, it was the source of the crystalline movement of life. It was the precursor to the original ball of starseed that exploded and created all that exists in our big-banging or, depending upon your cosmology, pulsating universe. And it flowed through me. I was connected with it as if by an immense shuddering optical fiber of not only light, but energy.

This was a pre-religious experience. Religion now seemed superfluous next to being in the presence of this source of life. Spirituality had become a limp representation of the fury and power of life. It was not awesome, it was awe itself. It was not godly but godding. It was not good, but was the way it was; it was the pure absolute that was not right, or loving, or benign, but was just the way it was—life alive.

Of <u>course</u> one loves all other living creatures. Of course one feels that everything is all right with creation. Of course we are all united. We are simply all part of the fire of life. If this source of energy that flows through us did not exist, neither would we. Love, spirituality, and peace follow from this experience as surely as one breath leads to another. No big deal. It is merely our nature.

Most astonishing of all, I could remember this connection from the past. It was flowing through me all the time. I had felt it earlier in my life, as a child. There seemed to be a dim memory of the immense glory of life from my infancy. Do we forget this incredible birthright as we age? It did not matter, for I knew what I was.

As the high point of the experience waned, I began to have experiences more common to other psychedelics. My open-eyed visual field meshed into hexagonal geometric patterns. When I looked at my own or at another's face, we seemed mythic, glowing, young, timeless, peaceful. Moving hands through the air trailed beaded radiant energy patterns. Spoken sentences took on multi-levels of understanding and cosmic punmanship. Most reported a levity, but not toward giggles but toward a deep, powerful peace. "This is the drug we never took," said one. "This is the natural state of human beings."

All of our group integrated smoothly back into ordinary reality, frequently remarking on the profundity of their experiences. Some reported no visual hallucinations like mine. One never went inside, for fear of engaging sad memories. Several stayed exterior to their internal processes and conversed and visited with each other during the whole episode. Some exhaustion was reported by each. I would recommend a day of complete rest for anyone who takes this drug.

A Rite of Passage into a New Vision

35 year-old male, graduate student, father of three §

My last experience with a substance in my search for the understanding of consciousness gave me a pleasant surprise. It was like a rite of passage, an initiation into a new vision of myself, my purpose, my mission, and my life. We all started with the setting up of an altar. Just the setting up of my shamanic power tools gave me a sense of anticipation of the power of the ritual with which I was about to be involved.

The experience with the substances was varied. With Adam I felt in that very familiar space that I have explored in the past. With 2CB I felt myself to be in a state of consciousness similar to the experiences I have had with magic mushrooms. At the end of the effects of Adam, and at the beginning of the effects of 2CB, I did a lot of work with what I call "junk." It was very powerful especially due to the fact that some issues concerning my mother arose into consciousness from a repressed space, and I was able to deal with them without fear and with compassion. Even though I still feel that I have more work to do in that area, the memories that came from the past were very powerful, and with my heart opened the way it was, I was able to see it with compassion and understanding.

After dealing with those issues, the rest of the evening was sheer pleasure for me. I felt my heart open like never before, and I would look at the rest of the people in the circle with a great amount of love and compassion. I was then channeling this love energy and I was really seeing everybody in a different light.

When we went around the circle, standing in each other's places,

---

§ *Set*: self-exploration; group and planetary healing and peace.
Setting: group of 12; weekend by the ocean; ritual circle.
Catalyst: 150 mg MDMA; 3.5 hours later, 20 mg 2CB.

this developed in me a deep empathetic understanding of every one of the people in the group. Even though my perceptions of the "space" of each person was different, with every one I felt a strong love connection and a great deal of compassion. That love feeling stayed with me during the rest of the night. It became clear that it was a turning point for me.

I reached the level in which the understanding of how we create reality was very solid, and in my inner world I realized that I had to stand on my own two feet for awhile; I said goodbye to my therapist, who was also present in this ceremony. It also became clear that to complete my ritual I had to give up my most "valuable" power object, my big crystal, the one that had been with me in the past. I also had to give it to the person who had guided me in my recent explorations, as a token of appreciation for the work that we had done together—and so I did.

I began that evening after the workshop to have the most amazing and powerful dreams that I have had in a long time, culminating on the fourth day with what I consider one of the most important "completion" dreams that I have experienced up to now. It had to do with the final letting go and separation from the esoteric group that I belonged to in the past. I had been trying to totally let go of any hold that they might still have on my consciousness.

In this dream I confronted one of the key persons in the group, who in the dream was acting as a sorcerer trying to separate a couple who were getting married. Something very unusual happened: while I was dreaming and confronting this person I found that I still could not beat her, but then I "woke up" and in the awake state of consciousness I found a feather I had collected that day when hiking, held it in my hands, closed my eyes, and was once again in my dream, in front of this person, but this time with the feather in my hand.

When I confronted this person with the power that the feather had given me, this negative entity disappeared, or I should say dissolved. I then fully awoke with a sense of lightness that I had never experienced before after a dream. It was as though a great weight had been removed from my body and my process of detachment from this group had reached a conclusion. I told my wife about it right away, and I felt happier and more connected with her than I had in a long time.

In all, the weekend was definitely a rite of passage: from heaviness to lightness, from prison to liberation, and from dependency to the realization that I have the power to guide my own destiny and to create my own reality.

Expressing Feelings Long Gone Unsaid

33 year-old male, depressed §

My main desire in using MDMA was as a means for franker, deeper communication with people I feel close to, but with whom this feeling is not often explored or expressed.

My experience with MDMA had two main components: the physical "high" and the interpersonal interactions. The latter was definitely the part of my MDMA experiences that were most strikingly different from anything I had ever experienced in my life, whether using drugs or not.

Physically, the rush that I felt as the drug took effect was similar to, but perhaps smoother than, my recollections of a limited number of trips on LSD, mushrooms, or other hallucinogens. In both MDMA experiments I first felt a gradual but steadily increasing light-headedness (a very pleasant high). This was joined within five or ten minutes by a strong feeling of warmth centered in my stomach and abdomen, but spreading out very evenly to my extremities. The headiness tapered off fairly early and became less noticeable as the sessions went on, but the sense of warmth throughout my body was quite pronounced.

After the initial physical effects established themselves, the interpersonal effects began to emerge. With the people in the first session whom I did not know very well, there were mainly very positive expressions of mutual pleasure and enjoyment of shared experience (we had just been together for six days on a vacation) and what seemed to be genuine desires for on-going friendships. These interactions could fall into the too-good-to-be-true category, because

---

§ *Set*: self-exploratory, enhanced communication.
Setting: at home, with small group, two therapists/guides.
Catalyst: two sessions, both 150 mg MDMA plus 50 mg MDMA; propranolol following first session.

they were overwhelmingly positive and hopeful, with almost no critical information exchanged. In short, these interactions were warm and to the point of being inspiring as long as I didn't examine them too carefully. Remembering them now, at some distance in time and space, I find that I am slightly suspicious of the depth and commitment of these exchanges.

With the people I knew well however, the intimacy and honesty that I felt being exchanged were unmatched in my experience. This is certainly the characteristic of MDMA that most impressed me on both occasions. The conversations, whether one-on-one or in the group of close friends, were close to the bone without causing defensive reactions. At least I felt this in myself. I was able to express feelings about myself and about my friends that had long gone unsaid; it felt very good and very sincere to be able to say these things.

Not everything said in the more intimate conversations was positive, either. Doubts and inadequacies, both past and present, were spoken of with relative ease and openness. Discussions were at a sustained level of seriousness that would ordinarily be difficult to maintain. There was very little drive to outdo each other with wit and one-upmanship; the conversations were to-the-point, with little hesitation or affectation. I didn't feel the need to tip-toe verbally, either; words came easily without the halting, searching style that I often notice in myself at times of attempted self-revelation.

This feeling was tempered by the strong feeling of shared concern that I felt. I seemed to be strongly and constantly aware of how much we all meant to one another. This feeling made further openness that much easier to achieve.

I reached a deeper understanding of my relationships with a small group of friends (those who participated in the session) and, by extension, a better awareness of how other people who know me well might perceive me. I also received a brief exposure to the personal belief systems of several people I respect very much, and this exposure led me to some thinking about my own philosophy.

The expressions of mutual concern and caring that came out between friends during the session definitely affected my general outlook for a short period of time (several weeks) after the session. I was somewhat less suspicious of other people's motives in general and I was more aware of expressing my feelings and my reactions to people around me. This outlook has faded as I have moved further in time from the session.

I think that the openness that emerged during the session has carried over into my day-to-day relationships; for a time after the session this was quite noticeable, but now it is more subtle and transitory.

I have been able to show more patience and tolerance in adjusting to unexpected and frustrating work circumstances. I think I am less prone to moodiness and temperamental silences, and I am more likely to confront difficult situations and to deal with them promptly. Again, however, these effects were more noticeable immediately after the session, and have been less so as time has passed.

"I Love You!" They Cried Out, Soundlessly

22 year-old male, college student §

I took the drug with four friends whom I had known for over six months and with whom I had been hanging out socially over the past few weeks.

We all took the drug and brought some music out to the recreation area, and we hung around and danced while we waited for the drug to take effect. After perhaps half an hour or a couple of us were definitely under the influence of the drug, and we started to touch each other and hug and squeeze. Soon someone suggested that we form a backrub daisy chain, and everyone thought that it was a good idea.

You could tell that people were really getting into the touching, for they were not only rubbing backs but also arms and heads, and they were giving big hugs, too. After a while, everyone turned around to give a backrub to the person who had been giving him or her one, and after that we decided to give foot massages to the person behind us.

We were doing this in a common area between the dorms, and other people frequently passed by us. Their reactions were interesting. Some made big circles in order not to get near us. Others were more curious and took a good look as they passed by. Many were sitting around watching us huddled in little groups. We were real open with what we were doing and we welcomed others to join our circle.

About seven people took up our offer. Some of them were also doing Adam; a few weren't on any drug as far as I knew.

After over an hour from when we took the drug, neither I nor my

---

§ *Set*: recreational.
Setting: college dorm recreation area, with 4–6 others.
Catalyst: 125 mg MDMA.

friend had yet got off. This was the first time that he had done any kind of psycho-active drug, and he seemed a little worried about not getting off. Everyone else was concerned and calm about us; they were keeping track of us without pestering us.

I wasn't too bothered. I've tripped on LSD several times and I knew that it sometimes took effect quickly and other times took longer. Nevertheless I thought that if I got up and became active that the drug might take effect more quickly. I left the group and ran around some and I came back to the group.

I returned to the circle, which actually was becoming less and less of a circle. The organization was breaking down, with some people touching the person behind them, others the person in front. Hands would reach across the circle in order to make contact with someone else. Some might find themselves massaging a calf and then ask whose calf they were massaging. Looks of love would be passed across the circle. Facial expressions reflected peace and comfort and pleasure and sheer heavenliness. "I love you," they cried out, soundlessly.

I'm sure that people who were looking on from nearby that this pile of squirming, sighing, and half-naked bodies had every appearance of an orgy. Most of the men had removed their shirts, and everyone's shoes were off for maximum available skin surface. How far would this go? The feeling was sensual but not—at least for me— sexual. I found myself completely aroused, yet not erect; whereas sexual touching often has the aim of raising the passions and of eventual intercourse, it seemed that touching was an end in itself. There was no idea of trying for gain.

The touching was pure communication. I like you. You are nice. This is fun. You are a human being whose friendship I value. I love you. So much was being said. Indeed, I don't think that this feeling precluded sexual feeling, for at times pairs would leave our circle, presumably to have sex alone. Now, after sharing the experience with others, I realize that it might very well have been that they just wanted to be alone with each other.

I stood up, and as soon as I did it became very clear that I was quite under the influence of the drug. As I stood, I shook a little, and I realized that everything felt differently. I was surprised because it wasn't like acid at all. There were no hallucinations nor was my mind scrambling from one thought to another. There was just this constant blissfulness, and a compassion for others. If everything looks different on LSD, then everything feels different on Adam. Not only does it effect the sense of touch, but is also effects the emotions, the yearnings, the feelings.

Two members of the group were hugging each other and I came up and started hugging them both. A couple of days ago I had been in one of their rooms, talking to her. She was down in spirits and as I left, I decided to give her a hug. I told her how hard it had been for me to do that, and how natural it was for me to do that now. I wanted to do that more often, I told her.

Everyone seemed to be telling others things that they had wanted to say for ages, yet never had the courage to spit out. One of them told me and another friend that of all the new students we were the two that he wanted to get to know. How nice to be told this. Another guy told his girlfriend that she was the first girl he had ever had romantic feelings for. The way he said this made it seem that he had been wanting to say it for a long time.

What was most unusual was that these deepest feelings were being expressed in public. It didn't matter if other people whom you didn't even know overheard. Indeed it was because of this that I heard all that I did.

Three of us stood there, hugging each other, massaging each others' backs, swaying. I was purring like a cat, constantly, and had been for some time. Faces lit up and eyes looked like stars. I kissed one member, lovingly and carefully, without lust. Wonderful. Then I kissed another man. The same. Not lovers' kisses, full of desire. Not mothers' kisses, clean and distant.

That's the first time I had ever kissed a male other than my father. Strange. I never felt even the slightest inclination to do so before. And it was so natural. Is love transitive? Does my love for the woman combined with her love for this man make me love him?

Could I have sexual relations with this man? Something I had never even conceived of before now loomed before me as a skitting possibility. How do I react to this possibility? Shortly afterward, I got into a conversation with someone who told me that the first time he did Adam he wound up in bed with his roommate. I saw how that could happen.

Another guy who had not taken the drug but who had been with us for some time came to me and started hugging me and rubbing me all over. Something was very strange, though. His hand was slowly inching towards my genitals. I twisted to prevent this and he continued working on me and he started going for me again. We repeated this several times. I really liked him touching me, but it seemed to me that he wanted something out of me and that made me uncomfortable. I didn't know him all that well, anyway.

It interested me that I had kissed a man but that I had really wanted to avoid this guy entirely. Then I realized that what had offended me about him was not that he was male but that he was being grasping and insensitive. If he had been on Adam he would have realized that I didn't want to fool around with him. I think he misunderstood the effects of the drug. He saw that we were being very physical and sensual and thought that we were being sexual, too. Or perhaps he was just hot for cock and was trying to take advantage of our condition. I later heard that he had made advances to many others.

During the days that followed I made great efforts to see the others I had done Adam with, hoping that what we had wasn't all gone. Oh, don't let it be a dream. I was especially eager to see my special friend, and after being unable to get in contact with her for a couple of days, I found myself getting very depressed. I longed for her.

It has been a week now since our Adam experience, and we have all gotten together several times. We've retained our ability to touch one another, by and large, and we have had massage parties of sorts at times. I've been able to hug other people much more easily and with fewer second thoughts than before. If I see someone I like and who is open, I give him or her a hug. I've realized how much all people like this kind of communication, despite their lack of any reaction, so long as they don't think that I'm hugging them in order to get something out of them. If one expects them to do anything in return, even something as little as hugging you back, then one is making a demand on them and they may feel uncomfortable.

I've found myself with much less sexual desire than before. It's as though the non-sexual touching has been an outlet for my sexual energies. This is a grand improvement, for I've found myself repeatedly driven to do things that I later regretted because of my sexual desire. Sex has also dominated my thoughts, and now I'm free to attend to things that I think are more important.

We Had All Just Been Born

25 year-old male, graduate student §

It is important to remember that what is being talked about here are the images and symbols of consciousness, and not necessarily the experience itself. The experience is felt before the mind attaches form, images, symbols, and structure in its functional attempt to communicate meaning. It is therefore my belief that some levels of consciousness precede some functional levels of mind and are simply beyond words. With this in mind, I would like to share that part of the group experience that I can talk about.

There were a number of very beautiful images of the journey. The first was shortly after the Adam blew through. The room was flushed with the richly warm gold light of the fire, and as my eyes flowed from person to person, the feeling came over me that I had been there before. I was in the nursery of a hospital and the room was filled with my fellow new-arrivals. It was as though we had all just been born and we were looking around to get a sense of each other and of the wonder of it all. The feeling of connectedness and love for everyone in the room was a very deep knowing. For the first time in my life I really felt like I belonged to the family of man.

Another image I had was that we were the survivors of a calamity at sea, clinging to a raft of timbers, being guided through the blackness of a raging storm by a captain who had gone mad with the loss of his vessel. This was the predominant theme of the journey that carried my fantasy images through the night. We were adrift on a sea of emotion, both collective and personal, and the raft was being tossed about more or less in accordance with the emotions being felt by the

§ *Set*: exploratory, group and planetary consciousness.
Setting: house by ocean; group of 12, guided ritual.
Catalyst: 150 mg MDMA; 3.5 hours later, 20 mg 2CB.

voyagers. There were couples clinging to each other out of fear, there was crying, some were moaning, others were consoling, as we collectively struggled with our souls on a cosmic voyage to Self.

The captain grappled with the staff (the talking staff being passed around) of our intergalactic raft, while spouting poems by Rumi like a mariner drunk with the Divine. He would inspire us not to despair in the midst of our personal and collective storms, and he brought light into the darkness. There were also periods of calm when the captain would soothe us with celestial music and send us off into the galaxies searching for Self: intergalactic cartographers exploring inner space. But the storm raged on into the darkness. The captain grasped the tiller with both hands, his hair swept back like a mad man, and he would sway around in a circular motion trying to steady the raft. His eyes would roll back into his head so that all was left were white orbs. Then he'd snap his head erect and fix his eyes on someone close by and say, "Get it?" The only thing missing was the salt spray, everything else was in there. It was an evening with Captain Ahab.

When Each is the Other, and Self as a Whole

35 year-old female, teacher §

In preparing for my first experience of Adam, I read some short reports of others' experiences and I asked questions about the differences between Adam and LSD, which I had taken twice in the previous six months. The three of us, with a guide, started to walk to a secluded beach that we had heard of.

About half an hour after taking the drug, I lay down on a blanket and began to shake. I surrendered to it peacefully, but I began to be torn between the realization that I was naked and that the sun was strong and I could get badly burned. I felt these thoughts holding me away from allowing the effects of the drug to take over. Then I sat up and put on my sweat suit and lay back down. At some point I found a palm-sized stone and held it in my right hand. I felt energy from it. I felt I understood that all of existence is energy—life.

I surrendered completely to the experience. I felt cold and I began to shake all over. A growing sense of freezing that started from behind my right ear and travelled across my throat to below the left ear, almost like the tingling sensation of dental anesthesia. I felt my jaw forced wide open to the point of pain in my jaw joints. I wondered later whether this was related to a tonsillectomy at the age of five. While in this strange, dark place of pain, I suddenly felt a very gentle touch on my right hand and I came back with a flooding sense of gratitude that our guide was there. It was as though I were being bathed in love and joy. I heard gentle music playing on the tape recorder near my head. Soon I was back completely in the immediacy of the present and the glorious surroundings of sea and rock and birds

---

§ *Set*: self-exploratory.
Setting: outdoors, beach, with three others, including a guide.
Catalyst: 150 mg MDMA.

and plants and sky and sun.

I remember sitting on the blanket, looking up and down the beach, watching the others on the rocks and under the waterfall, playing together, and I thought, "Why am I sitting here by myself? Why am I not included?" Then I got up and went over to the rocks, but the others had left. I enjoyed being close to the water, I loved the feel of the rocks and the sense of connectedness. I was aware of time being, as it were, timeless. I had no sense of needing to do anything. I felt the freedom to simply respond to any urge that occurred. When I wished to join the others, I did so. When I wished to be alone, I was so.

After awhile I was aware that our guide and E were lying side by side not far from me. E seemed very sad. I watched them for some time and wondered whether to confront E, and finally I decided to do so. After a while the guide left us alone. Gradually E got closer and I began to feel almost claustrophobic, but without panic, which would have been my reaction without the drug. I quietly disengaged and I walked away feeling clear that I could leave because I wanted to, without having either to reassure the other or battle the other, or myself. I could simple separate myself from another; I did not have to separate myself from myself, as I have so often in the past.

I moved away from the rocks at the other end of the beach, to where I had last seen the guide. He had climbed up onto a rock above the waves, which I found was part of a stone bridge. I moved and sat on the bridge itself with my legs spread so that the water seemed to pound between them. I felt and exulted in the force of the sea pounding through me, into me, a part of me. I was the sea, I was me, I was both, and I was the rock. As I described this several times during the following week I spoke of the femaleness of the sea. I felt myself as the rock being penetrated by the sea—surrendering to that powerful and exultant, sexual, male/female union of rock and sea, when the distinction of male and female seemed blurred, when each is the other and the self as a whole.

The next morning I wrote: "I awoke this morning with images of male genitals of different sizes and shapes. I thought about our guide and E, and of how different they are. I became aware of myself, of my femaleness and the feeling of tenderness and curiosity about the male. I suddenly felt that my homosexuality had been a search for understanding and acceptance of the femaleness of myself. I felt so at ease yesterday with nakedness—my own and others'. I looked at our friends' bodies, which were so very like an ancient fertility or earth goddess. The great round shapes, breasts, stomachs, hips, all firm as though she were made of wonderful fruits, not soft, but ripe, glorious."

I enjoyed gazing at D's body and what she was doing with it. The top of her body was so thin and young and her belly was large and round as though she were pregnant. Her head reached forward, lips pursed in an almost monkey expression. Her evident joy—no, immediacy—being totally where she was; and the feeling I had was that she was glad about the experience. I became aware of feeling repulsed by E but at the same time compassionate. I had no desire to cuddle close to him and I had no sense of fear or anger when he evidently wanted me closer to him. I could allow his caresses and his kissing my brow—not an unpleasant sensation—and then easily, and without hurting him, drift away.

All day my cold seemed gone, no stuffiness, no coughing, no pain in my throat or chest. The next day my cold came back with a worrisome sharp pain in my chest, but that lasted for only half a day. The effect of the drug was evident to me for about five days, giving me the feeling of being more open and connected with people and with nature than I usually feel. The greatest shift in myself is in my attitude towards the understanding and the appreciation of the men around me.

A Very Deep Kundalini Experience

32 year-old male, professional §

I took 150 plus 63 mg Adam. While lying down to wait for the effect I did not feel well, rather depressed. The effect began after forty minutes, and after one hour I wanted to leave my cave, being attracted by other people of our group who walked happily along the beach. I felt very attracted by the sand as part of Mother Earth, and I sat for a long time pouring sand all over my body like a snake or a crab, sideways. Slowly people came together and a long period of close and intimate contact began.

I felt totally safe, self-confident, really identified with my Buddha nature and relating to the very same nature in other people. That's how God created us! Then M. had a kundalini episode that frightened me initially very much; there was so much openness that, her fear and my fear melted and our connection increased. I started clenching my jaws, which was obviously more than a drug effect and was in fact a dramatization of my usual way of dealing with my fear. I found that sucking a woman's breast or kissing released the clenching immediately so I did that a lot with great delight.

Coming down was quite difficult in the next three days. I could observe in detail how the closing up of my openness was related to a series of subtle fear reactions starting from my fear with M's kundalini experience. I again found myself very depressed, at the same time observing more clearly the process of getting depressed and seeing new perspectives with which to deal with it: trying to stay open and talk without the drug—very simple, very difficult.

A week later I did a much more internalized trip. I was lying on

---

§ *Set*: therapeutic, self-exploration.
Setting: outdoors and inside, with friends/sitters in small group.
Catalyst: 150–200 mg MDMA.

my blanket, rocking gently and becoming identified with my happy self, which was talking and teaching my depressed self. I was supported by this very gentle, floating guitar music. I could show to my depressed self that there have been happy times in my mother's womb (even though my mother didn't want the pregnancy), especially during the latter stages of the pregnancy. We—my two selves—experienced being gently carried around on vacations in Lausanne: I could see the sea and the beach promenade (I must check with my mother to see whether she had been there one or two months before my birth!). I tenderly encouraged my depressed self, and I laughed with it, and showed a lot of love to it.

At the same time my right arm shook for about two hours in a steady kundalini rhythm that felt just wonderful! Finally my shaking right hand banged for a long time against my sixth chakra, then against the seventh, causing flashes of lightning within my head. This was the first kundalini experience of my life, and a whole new perspective of looking at tensions and symptoms opened up. My right arm became paralyzed when my father died, and my psychoanalyst could not really clear up the symptom.

Then I needed more dramatic music, "Shakti," by John McLaughlin, and I was gently born. A wonderful period of contact began. The coming-down was less difficult because my happy self did some preparatory work for that and because the session had come to a completion after going through some more important work.

Three days later I went into another Adam experience with a strong orientation of "I want to go further with that kudalini experience." For a long time I repeatedly played "Shakti," and again I experienced a lot of shaking. I could study very clearly the inhibiting effect of thinking and planning on the spontaneous unfolding of that shaking life force. I got some very clear insights into my actual relationships and I found the courage to clear them up. Also I understood that the paralysis of my arm was an attempt to suppress shaking as an expression of all the tensions and contradictory feelings in that period, as well as other physical symptoms, especially in the lower back. I could see that the effect of Adam decreases when taken too often in a short period of time and that the side effects increase (headaches).

The next day I had my last breathing session in our workshop: it was the most important and intense session I had ever had—a very deep kundalini experience. I see Adam as a perfect preparation for that non-drug experience and I am very grateful for that.

Mother Earth Communicated Her Grounded Presence

37 year-old married woman §

I came into the group feeling extremely centered, grounded. A week of meditation and solitude, connecting with nature, had set the stage for what became a very rewarding, enriching experience. All of my fears never materialized, they were only fears created in the mind of ego.

My prayer to Mother Earth was answered from the start. Mother Earth communicated her powerful message of grounded presence, deeply penetrating through to my own core of Being. Now matter how expansive the mind became, Mother Earth held on to me, keeping the connection and the agreement we made together, no matter how much I wanted to soar, to fly off into realms unknown. I had agreed to be fully present and mindful, to be open to others' experiences, and to openly share with my heart their journeys.

When we sang each others' names, I began to truly touch the heart of each and every soul whose name we called out. Even now I find myself singing out these names, which makes my heart sing of love and respect for the unique beauty and charm that each person shared with me. How I love each and everyone so dearly! While writing this I feel a sense of loss—I miss their presence. But when I sing out their names, they are magically present and real.

Never have I felt so much love and joy with a group. I wanted to express this, but how? My heart was so open, drinking in the rich energy that filled the room. I humbled myself over each person's place, bowing down to their magnificent radiant Light. Mother Earth guided me, urging me to serve the group as well as my heart commanded.

---

§ *Set*: self-exploration; group and planetary consciousness.
Setting: group of 12, guided ceremonial.
Catalyst: 150 mg MDMA plus 50 mg 2CB.

There were times when we were often on our own individual journeys of self-exploration. I thought about my family and friends. I was struck by how much love they have for me. I had to honor that somehow. I need to learn to be more accepting, more forgiving of their shortcomings, for the only experience I can truly share with them is one of complete abiding trust and respect for each and every one of them. They have chosen their own paths to individuation and union with God; mine is not to question these paths but to honor them. It doesn't matter that I may not always understand what they do or why.

When love pours forth from within me like the incessant waves of the eternal sea, I know that Love is the only source of power—nothing else is as real or as true as this power to love. And when it touches others, then I feel closest to the Divine Spirit—my heart soars to tremendous heights and depths.

I thought deeply of my husband, of how much my love for him is blessed by Divine Will. All issues, difficulties between us seemed insignificant when in touch with the power of this love. I was struck by the realization that our destinies lie in the all-knowing presence of God. No matter what direction our realization takes us in, it is still within God's universal plan. I must learn to let go and let this plan unfold as it should, regardless of the outcome. My mission is to be open to the lessons we are learning from one another and to remain unconditionally supportive of our individual goals. No matter what happens, our love will continue to deepen and to expand, for that is our truth!

The high point came quite unexpectedly during the morning's sharing ritual. I didn't realize how the ecstasy from within grew to unknown dimensions. Once again I could not contain all the love and joy I felt for everyone. Giving expression to this in the form of dancing, singing, touching, hugging, etc., brought the intensity of feelings to an all time high.

I Meet the Feminine Half of Myself

26 year-old male, programmer, poet §

One of the things I wanted to work on was finding the inner feminine in me, and as an adjunct to that, the releasing of a lover into the new place of friend only. I began thinking of that intention as I began to feel completely involved in the drug and had an experience of traveling through many of the eight planes of experiencing, to what I felt was in the fifth plane. I felt as if I were taken into a red pyramid where I met the feminine half of myself, and I felt as if the meal were a ritual symbolic of me accepting her and of her accepting me—a marriage on some level of me with her.

After this ceremony I felt as if I were taken back to my body, where I remembered about what had happened and tried out my new person by remembering several of the women I know and by visualizing myself being with them from this new place. I noticed that I felt less anxiety and fewer demands on myself and on them.

After several hours we ingested the second substance. I remember feeling a bit of anxiety about where it might take me.

I wanted to work on healing a situation that often turns unpleasant for me; it happens in the evening after I have come home alone and have no plans for the evening. I start to feel closed off and unhappy, often giving into depression and going to bed to sleep and avoid my feelings. Again I felt the presence of a dark spot in me, yet even as I tried to send it light I felt as if I was unable to reach it at this time. I remember wondering if this meant that I would need to go through some more depression and unhappiness, and I remember not wanting to do that. I felt surprised that I was unable to heal that place.

---

§ *Set*: therapeutic (for depression); group and planetary consciousness. *Setting*: home by ocean, guided ceremony, 12 experienced travellers. *Catalyst*: 150 mg MDMA; 4 hours later, 20 mg 2CB.

Another issue I worked on somewhat was work. I have been hitting obstacles in work and last week I was unable to go through them. The only answer I could get for myself was that I needed to bring more of myself to work. While at the ruby pyramid I thought of the situation, and the answer seemed to be that I must bring my inner-wife along to work.

At one point we went out and looked at the stars; that was a wonderful experience. Before I had always felt sort of alone and apart when looking up at the stars, but this time I felt an aliveness and a belonging to those vast distances. That was a wonderful feeling.

I had some interesting perceptions of reality. At one point one of the women was sitting at the fire place and I wanted to reach out to her. I noticed that as my thoughts about it changed, so did my perceptions of the situation: when I thought she wouldn't like it, I felt closed in and dark and unable to move, and when that passed and I realized that I didn't know what she wanted unless I did it, I felt an opening. It seemed as if each thought I had and each action I took changed the reality of the situation.

One of the most important parts for me was going to the sea the following morning after everyone was awake. I noticed that there were so many living things in the grasses on the way to the sea. Everything seemed alive.

I wanted to find something on the ocean to take back to remind me of the journey. I realized I could not will that to happen, that something would have to choose me, and that it had already been decided—regardless of how I thought or how I acted. I realized that I might find nothing, and that that would have to be OK with me. On the way back up the hill I leaned over and picked up a piece of driftwood, the leaning coming by itself without any thought.

At one point I wandered out to the sea and stood on the edge. I recalled the place I had been during the past week of wondering whether I really wanted to live and of realizing that I could simply swim into the sea and vanish into the ocean. It felt as if that would be similar to my death, when it comes to that, that death is a being swallowed up into something greater. I felt as if it was not right for me to do that (there is a very important distinction: there was no wrongness about it, it's just that that act would not have been right). As I stood I realized that if I chose to return that I would have to take responsibility for my life, that I would have to live differently, that I would have to stand for myself. Again, after a time, I made the decision and walked up the hill.

After my choice at the ocean and walking along the beach to go back, I picked up a rock. I held it in my hands and poured into it all of my feelings of being alone and being depressed and all of my lack of aliveness, and I hurled it far out into the ocean.

Before leaving for the ocean I didn't feel a sense of fullness or particularly good. I wondered if I would go away from the session feeling scattered and alone. After coming back and sharing the meal and passing the staff, I felt a sense of well-being, and I felt this as I started to connect with people and talk with them in a new way.

Driving back into the city I had a vision of our society as like the freeway, so many people hurtling forward in cars down this tiny lane, except that it seemed in the vision that we ended up in a heap of wrecked automobiles.

I wonder about the time we live in, about the healing work that we did on the planet. There seems to be such a need for light here. Lately I have had a different sense of what reincarnation means: it means that I will be here on the earth again in the future. Sometimes I feel as if my task here is to find that healing power that was found everywhere on earth at one time in myself, and let that power be in my heart and let it go forth from me to everyone.

Today, the day after the session, I have stayed home. I felt I needed to assimilate what has happened. I feel differently. I feel I can stand on my own two feet. I feel I can stand tall. I feel I can speak with my own voice. I notice that in the past I would consider staying home a sign of weakness, and that today I see it as a sign of being true to my process, to my self.

What else is important? I realized in the middle of the session that I had been wrong about how I saw my relationships to people. I used to feel that I must be able to be completely alone to be whole/happy. Maybe that was the cause of much of my depression. Because I experienced that I am connected with people, even when I go within to myself, somehow they are a part of me, and I am involved in giving and receiving with them. I experienced that it is OK to be connected with people, that we flow in and out of each other's lives for a reason, and that it is all right to do this, that it is in the scheme of things. I experienced that the person who no longer wants to be lovers with me is strongly connected with me for now, and that this next phase is as important and as loving as the first phases.

When I go within now I experience myself in a new sort of wholeness and completeness, yet even as I do that I feel my connections with others more strongly. It is almost as though the more I fill up the more I connect, the more I accept the connections.

Ocean Vastness Enters Me

36 year-old female, photographer, scientist §

Taking the Adam. Then drumming for the journey. That was good. It was a way to structure the time, something to focus on. I was aware of beginnings of visual changes toward the end of the drumming. After the drumming was over I lay down and paid attention to my breathing without trying to do anything about it. I felt a beginning of melting and expansion. It was so easy now to let light and awareness and energy move through places in my neck and shoulders that have been painfully blocked recently. There were layers of opening, and a sense of the heart expanding and opening. It was a sacred journey that we were all on together.

I thought of various people in my life—co-workers, friends, etc. I sent love to each of them. Then there was more expansion and I sent love farther and farther out. I was aware of gratitude towards my parents. I sent love to them. I let them know that their jobs as parents were complete. They were free to die, or to live on a while as my friends. I released my attachment to them. I saw that most people are doing the best they know how as parents, even Reagan. It's just that their knowledge, and my own, are so limited most of the time.

I expanded even more. I realized that I don't have to use my mind to direct the light and love. All I have to do is be an open channel. The light has a wisdom of its own. It is awesome to be part of this group channel, to bring light into the earth.

More opening occurred. I went further than I've ever gone before. Somewhere along here my guide suggested that we all hold hands. I was aware of the vastness of the ocean out to my left. I felt that

§ *Set*: exploratory, group and planetary consciousness.
Setting: home by ocean, guided group of 12 experienced travellers.
Catalyst: 150 mg MDMA; 4 hours later, 20 mg 2CB.

vastness enter me. I don'tremember how, but I became aware of an image of nuclear war and of environmental destruction. I thought of scientists. Then I felt as though a slimy, black ooze monster were coming up out of the ocean and engulfing me from the left side. I felt terror, chaos. I felt I was out of control and that I was being consumed and drowned by something chaotic and evil. I seemed to be inside and outside. I felt as if I were losing it completely. The experience wasn't totally new. I had a sense I'd been there before, perhaps in other psychedelic sessions.

Then I remembered that I wasn't alone, so I rolled over onto my left side and I held my guide's hand with both of my hands. The chaos subsided and I rolled again onto my back. I realized that the blackness had gotten me because I as a scientist felt some guilt about the destruction of the earth. I saw the needs of the scientists—they've been idealized, made into high priests. Now they are being seen as the bad guys. They are hurt, bewildered, and angry, and they need our compassion.

I felt the same stuff come at me again, but this time I let it through. What came in through me, as water woman, was passed on through the group and sent up the chimney in the consuming fire through the fire man.

Then I rolled over onto my stomach and I felt the reverse flow. Light-fire was coming down the chimney and was cleansing and purifying and washing all the junk into the ocean. I felt good to let it go out of my right side. Through all of this feeling I experienced the reality of the subtle realms of being; and they were as real as the physical, perceptual, emotional, and mental realms.

Later I became aware that I was coming down more, and I felt myself open and close to the flow of light and love. I looked around at the group, and I saw such warmth of human "being," and the candlelight and fire-light. I exchanged looks and smiles with various people. I felt much love for our camp director-guide, and I appreciated his sharing of his experience of the reality of these non-ordinary realms. The dancing we did in each other's places was wonderful. I strongly felt each person's being in his or her place. I got to know more of what it was like to be who they are, and I felt that each person was an aspect of myself. It was so amazing to be human.

At some time during the night I saw our guide as an elder who was passing on his wisdom to us; this whole thing was a giveaway. I saw inner images of his body growing older, becoming a corpse, then a skeleton with teeth falling out. All of this seemed exactly as it should be. I had an awesome sense of the relation of the finite to the infinite, of time to eternity, of mortality to immortality. Then I saw how near I was to the middle of my life and, while I am still looking ahead and taking in more, I am also beginning to turn back and share and give away. I felt very good to be aware of this.

After drinking the orange juice with the 2CB in it, I lay there wondering what would happen next. I was a little apprehensive, but I decided to just trust my guide's decision.

Then I began to feel vaguely uncomfortable. Partly I was just very tired from the strenuous afternoon and early evening. Soon I became aware of some imagery, aqua lightning bolts moving inside a dark human form, moving through the torso and limbs. I felt like I was losing the clarity of the earlier part of the evening. I didn't like what I was feeling. I don't have much sense now of the order of the following experiences, so I'll just list them as I think of them.

I felt physical and emotional pain, and the overstress of the body. I felt that my lifestyle was too stressful and I needed to change. Many images of driving fast on freeways, and I felt a lot of fear that I had not been aware of.

I heard other people moaning and I didn't like it. I thought critically of them and of myself, that I shouldn't be in such a negative place, that it is a childish attention-getting manipulation. I wanted to ask my guide to help me process all that was going on, but I thought that it was not OK to ask for individual attention in the group setting. I was scared, angry, confused. Only when I was really wanting to die did D reach over and touch me. That helped.

I felt a lot of anger about men and women as the night went on. I talked with T some. I cried out some of the pain I'd been in. People so much idealize the feminine in nature and so mistreat it in female humans. It was good to have T hold me as I cried. I didn't care that I was being a distraction for others. Later, I began to feel that I might be able to sleep.

When I awoke it was light. I was still angry and I was afraid to express it. I went into the bathroom and cried for awhile. I wanted to leave. I couldn't just lie in my space. I packed up all my stuff, not sure whether I'd leave or stay. I probably would have left angry or suicidal if the "Om Namah Shivah" chant hadn't been put on. That created an impersonal space that I could tolerate.

I went back to the beach. It was good to have my power spot to go to. I was glad to find that the spiral I had drawn in the sand was still there. I had with me the prayer arrow I'd made from a reed, feathers, and seaweed. I was glad to have that, too. Very simply and directly I asked for help transforming my relationship with the guide. I went and put the prayer arrow in the sand and I watched the waves wash around it.

I walked along the beach, and I felt stronger and less afraid and more balanced. I saw the guide communing with the ocean, and I felt more ready to meet him.

I climbed up and waited by the house. After the guide returned he came directly to me and greeted me. I felt that something had cleared. We were looking at each other more clearly. His greeting and hug were a real gift and a healing. After that I was able to talk with people. The morning breakfast and sharing were good. I felt that I had found a new inner strength.

In the week since, the experience has come and gone a few times. But basically I feel both stronger and more gentle and open. And I am more compassionate with myself and with other people.

Guidelines for the Sacramental Use of Empathogenic Substances

by Ralph Metzner with Padma Catell

The following guidelines have been compiled from the collective experience of about twenty or thirty therapists who have used these substances in their work, and who have formulated their methods based on their observation of hundreds of individual sessions. While there is by no means uniformity of approach among the different practitioners, the guidelines offered here do represent a kind of distillation of methods that have proven their efficacy. These guidelines should not in any way be construed as encouraging the use of illegal substances; rather they are applicable to any state of heightened empathic awareness, regardless of how the state is generated.

Although we realize that the use of MDMA and other drugs of this family occurs most frequently in what might be called a hedonistic or recreational context, with no particular therapeutic or spiritual purpose in mind, these types of sessions will not be discussed here. It is the belief of the present authors, and of the therapists and individuals represented in this book, that such occasional recreational use, while probably less harmful than the regular use of alcohol or tobacco, does not have the intrinsic interest and healing potential that guided, intentional, therapeutic, and sacramental use has. Specifics of this approach will be described under the headings of *Preparation and Set, Alchemical Catalysts, Setting and Context, Process and Method in Individual Sessions, Ritual Structure in Group Sessions, and Re-entry and Follow-up Factors.*

Preparation and Set

The single most important foundation for a beneficial experience is intention or purpose. One should ask oneself, and discuss with the therapist or guide, "What is my purpose in entering into this altered state of awareness?" Typically, people approach the experience with fundamental existential and spiritual questions, such as, "Who am I?" or "What is my Purpose in Life?" or "What is the Next Step in my Spiritual of Life Path?"

These are questions that all seekers have, and it is natural to want to ask them in the course of an encounter with one's sources of inner wisdom. In addition there may be more personal and therapeutic questions. These may include questions concerning physical illness, traumatic or conflicted experiences from the past, including early childhood and birth, and questions concerning imbalanced or unsatisfactory relationships with others, usually those closest to us, particularly parents, spouses, lovers, children, family and friends. It is not uncommon for individuals to spend major portions of the experience reviewing and trying to understand and heal interpersonal relationships.

Other kinds of issues people have explored are concerns regarding work and career, questions about creative expression or blocks, and questions concerning collective and global issues. Some therapists and guides encourage the person to make a written list of intentions, which can then be reviewed just prior to or even during the session, and perhaps recorded to assist recollection. Some people prefer to declare an intention to explore certain areas or topics, rather than posing questions. In either approach, it is a good practice to submit the questions and intentions to one's own higher knowing just prior to ingestion. In that way one is not too intent on problem solving, which could lead to a more limited view, rather than an openness to whatever unfolds which will most likely contain the answers to one's questions, even including those not asked but implied.

If the experience is the first one with a particular substance, it is also useful to discuss with the guide or therapist any fears one might have concerning the drug, and any other expectations, which may be based on one's past history or what one has heard from other people.

The question of sexual feelings and sexual expression between the people present should be raised before the session begins. If the relationship is a professional one, then the principle of no sexual contact should be discussed and affirmed. If the people are friends who are not lovers, their feelings for each other should be stated and clarified. They will be in a state of extraordinarily heightened emotional intimacy for several hours. This state facilitates an unusual degree of access to fears, concerns and frustrations in the area of intimacy. It is not advisable to use this heightened, open-state for the initiation of an ordinary sexual encounter. Even if the guide and the voyager are married or lovers, it is probably best to postpone actual sexual contact to the latter part of the experience because sexual contact will tend to distract from the exploration of other areas.

If two individuals who are lovers, and are experienced with empathogenic substances, wish to use a conjoint session to intentionally explore deeper levels of emotional and sexual and spiritual intimacy, this is certainly a state in which tantric and taoist eroticism, which is non-striving, non-craving, and non-possessive, can be experienced. Several of the accounts in this book testify to the extraordinary tactile sensitivity and sensuousness of the MDMA experience. But for the more usual kind of session, where someone is being initiated into this heightened awareness for the first time for purposes of psychospiritual awakening, an agreement or understanding of no sexual contact is preferable. As part of the discussion around this, it is important to also agree that the physical touch of a hand on the heart, the shoulder, the head or the hand, can be an important source of support and encouragement and that this represents empathy or compassion, but not sexual interest.

Another important part of the preparation, usually done just before the session, as part of the discussion of intention and purpose, is to practice a meditation with which one is familiar, or a basic relaxation procedure, so that one can enter into the enhanced state from a baseline that is already somewhat clear, centered, and free from distracting everyday concerns. Some people like to read, or have read to them, a favorite passage from a personally meaningful text, such as a chosen prayer, a beautiful poem, a passage from the *Course in Miracles*, or similar inspirational writings. For some people the prayer or meditation might include the specific invocation of a beloved guru or teacher and/or the invocation of a particular deity or guardian spirit. People have had extraordinarily powerful experiences with such figures as the Great Goddess, Jesus, Shiva, or American Indian Spirit Beings. Such prayers and invocations should of course not be imposed by the guide or therapist, but rather should come out of the individual's own practice.

Some people familiar with shamanic practices and rituals like to bring "power objects," such as crystals or feathers or any object that has been psychically charged, to the session. Some others, especially if wanting to explore relationship issues, might bring photographs of parents or family to contemplate, or photographs of themselves as children to activate childhood memories. Finally, it is recommended that one fast for at least six hours (usually with juices), or for anywhere from one to several days beforehand, so a full stomach does not reduce the substance's effect and also as part of a general psychic and physical purification. This also will tend to make the journey more productive and pleasant.

Alchemical Catalysts

Since the goal of alchemy was the transformation of consciousness, symbolized in the chemical and biological transmutations taking place within the human body, the physical substrate of consciousness, the *prima materia*, it is appropriate to call these chemical substances, ones that facilitate a transformative response, "alchemical catalysts." The discussion here is limited to the catalysts that are generally agreed to have primarily empathogenic effects, and will not address other hallucinogenics such as LSD, psilocybin or mescaline. For more extensive information on the botany, chemistry and pharmacology of MDMA the reader is referred to *Ecstasy: The Complete Guide* (Holland, 2001) and to the MAPS website, which has bibliographies on all the current research with these substances (www.MAPS.org).

The compounds of this empathogen (or entactogen) class that have been used in the accounts in this book include MDMA and 2CB (a very small number of experiences also included ketamine). Earlier work done in the 1970s by the Chilean psychiatrist Claudio Naranjo, M.D., also studied MDA and MMDA—although these variants have disappeared from both research and underground use. Many other molecules have been synthesized and found to be psychoactive, but none has attained the widespread attention that MDMA has. Chemically they are referred to as phenethylamines; and their chemical synthesis is described in Alexander Shulgin's uniquely eccentric compendium *PIHKAL—Phenethylamines I Have Known and Loved* (Shulgin & Shulgin, 1991).

Botanically, some of these compounds are found in the volatile oils of certain plants, including nutmeg and mace. Structurally, they resemble dopamine, a neurotransmitter; mescaline, a potent hallucinogen; and amphetamine, a stimulant. Their psychological effects are not unlike a blend of mescaline and amphetamine, although less hallucinogenic than the former, and less stimulating than the latter.

There is great individual variation in sensitivity to these substances; so one should at all times proceed with caution. One should always begin with a lower dose, and only gradually, if desired, progress to higher amounts.

MDMA is psychoactive in dosages of 50 mg to 250 mg; 150 mg is the usual effective dose for the average adult. It is shorter-acting than MDA, which had some popular use in the 1960s in the dance-scene. MDMA usually lasts three to four hours; and at the higher dosages has some amphetamine-like side-effects, such as muscular tremor, and jaw-clenching. Onset of pharmacologic effects usually occurs within 20 to 30 minutes after ingestion, and there is a transient moderate rise in blood pressure and pulse rate. Subjectively there is a rise in feelings of bodily heat, greatly increased attention and alertness, and after some time, bodily relaxation and ease.

Another chemical sometimes used in the present series of studies is 2CB. This is more potent (active at lower doses) than MDMA, being active in some people at 5–15 mg, with 20–25 mg as the recommended maximum dose. Energy tremors, jaw-clenching, heat, and an increase in blood pressure are the type of stimulant side-effects usually seen. Like MDMA, 2CB is empathogenic, although it appears to be somewhat more body-oriented, and also to have some mild visual effects, similar to mescaline. Some of the therapists and researchers cited in this book experimented with MDMA followed by 2CB three to four hours later. This basically serves to extend the empathogenic experience by the same amount of time. Some of the group experiences reported in this volume also used this combination.

Many of the side-effects of these substances are basically due to the response to their amphetamine-like stimulant action. These side-effects are very much dose-dependent. Most frequently noticed are jaw-clenching and fine to gross muscular tremors. Many people have found that a calcium-magnesium supplement (300–500 mg), taken just before, during, or after ingestion of the MDMA, can greatly reduce the intensity of these side-effects, or eliminate them altogether. There is usually complete loss of appetite during the duration of the experience (as is common for amphetamines) and even for a few hours afterwards. There may be fatigue or depressed mood the next day, perhaps partly due to the reduced food intake and to a depletion of stored serotonin. Vitamin and mineral supplements are recommended before and after the experience. Plenty of water should be consumed and available at all times, since there may be considerable dehydration. After the experience, some people take 500 mg of tryptophan, an amino acid, to help them sleep. Some take 100 mg of 5-HTP to decrease the depressive after-symptoms.

Contraindications for the use of these substances (which are, it must be remembered, relatively unresearched pharmacologically), include heart-disease or high blood pressure, history of psychosis, hypoglycemia and diabetes, seizure disorders, and of course pregnancy, as with any drug. When in doubt, one's physician should always be consulted.

It should always be remembered that these substances produce an intense though transient altered state of awareness. Although one's perception of everyday reality is not appreciably altered with the empathogens (unlike the hallucinogens like LSD), one's emotional response to reality is greatly amplified. Thus, although technically a person may be able to walk around, converse, or even drive an automobile during these states, this is obviously not desirable because the heightened state of emotional sensitivity could interfere with one's reactions. These tasks would take one away from the interior exploration of the psyche, which is after all the main point of the experience.

Setting and Context

Generally, the preferred setting for sessions in the therapeutic-sacramental mode is a serene, simple, comfortable room, in which the client, or voyager, can recline or lie down, and the therapist or guide can sit nearby. One's clothes should be loose and comfortable, and a blanket should be available in case of transient episodes of chilling.

It is best if there is access to, or proximity to, the elements of nature: a fire in a fireplace serves as a reminder of the alchemical fires of inner purification, and the life-preserving fire of Spirit. Fresh water to drink, and proximity to a stream or ocean, reminds us of the watery origins of our life. There should be access to fresh air, so one can experience the unutterable preciousness and sweetness of the breath of life. Earth and its natural forms—soil, plants, trees, rocks, wood—should also be close to the touch. Trees or plants in or near the room of the session make wonderful companions. Crystals or other stones may be held and contemplated.

The music played, usually selected and changed by the guide or sitter, can have a profound effect on consciousness. Entire therapeutic processes, or shamanic journeys, can be induced using certain musical selections. Generally, the therapists and individuals working with MDMA and other empathogens have found the serene, peaceful, meditative music sometimes referred to as "inner space" music, to be most valuable during these experiences. For most people fast or highly complex music seems irritating and too difficult to follow. Composers such as Kitaro, Vangelis, Deuter, Schoener, Paul Winter, and the slower baroque music of Bach or Vivaldi have become favorites of many users of empathogens. Simple gongs, bells and chimes can also be pleasing and centering during such experiences, whether one plays them or merely listens to them.

The attitude and behavior of the guide or sitter during the session is of course extremely influential; this role should be undertaken with integrity and sensitivity. If the guide is the person's therapist, then they have a therapeutic agreement to explore any areas of concern. If the sitter is a friend or even partner, it is best to have a clear agreement and understanding determined before the session, as to what the role of the guide should be. Most people prefer to, and are perfectly able to, do their own best therapy while in these states. They want the sitter merely to be there meditating quietly, perhaps changing recorded music, listening and recording the remarks of the voyager, providing water, encouragement, and reassurance if needed. Intense explorations of certain issues, for example relationships, sexuality, birth trauma or the like, should only be undertaken by prior agreement, or at the specific request of the voyager and ideally with a therapist who is experienced in this type of work.

In the state of emotional openness during these experiences, it can be easy for the voyager to become caught up in an analytical, verbal mode, perhaps in a discussion with the guide, that can take him or her away from the inner experience of heart-center awareness. Even if the interpersonal interaction between the two is warm, affectionate and trustful, it can still be a distraction from the deeper intrapsychic awareness that is possible when attention is primarily focussed inward. These shifts in attention can be subtle and elusive. The wise guide will watch for signs of when the voyager is losing his or her connection to the deep source within, and will help to refocus attention toward that source.

Process and Method in Individual Sessions.

Legally sanctioned access to MDMA-assisted therapy is currently unavailable except in a very small number of approved research projects. For this reason we will not enter into a discussion of the processes and methods of individual therapy assisted by empathogens. The MAPS website has links to the work of Michael and Annie Mithoefer in North Carolina, who are currently conducting studies in the use of MDMA in psychotherapy with PTSD, and in the course of that work, are training some therapists and student-therapists in their methods. We strongly believe (and it should go without saying) that <u>no therapist should consider administering or guiding a session with these substances who has not had personal experiences with those substances.</u>

The present guidelines are based on the experiences of therapists who have used these substances in their work when and where this was possible. A very valuable source of information and guidance about this kind of work is the book by Myron Stolaroff—*The Secret Chief*, about the pioneering work of a pseudonymous underground psychotherapist who used these catalysts in his work over a twenty year period with remarkable effectiveness. The book was republished in 2005 in a new edition, *The Secret Chief Revealed* (Stolaroff, 2005) in which the actual name—Leo Zeff—of the now deceased therapist was published. It would be my guess that Leo Zeff personally trained and initiated probably several dozen psychotherapists (myself among them—RM) in his spiritually and psychologically profound methods of amplified psychotherapy. The remainder of this section will merely give a few suggestions, primarily for the use of the individual undergoing the experience.

The questions, purposes, or agenda brought to the session, as discussed above under *Preparation and Set*, will basically set the tone of the experience. Whatever unfolds during the experience will be, in a sense, an answer to those questions (even although this may not become apparent until much later). Many of the therapists from whom these findings were obtained, suggest to the voyager to go first as far and deeply within as they can, to the core or ground of being, to their Highest Self, or give similar directions. From this place of total centeredness, compassion and insight, one can review and analyze the usual problems and questions of one's life. It is not uncommon for people to experience, and report to the therapist, that all their questions and problems have been dissolved in the all-embracing love and compassion that they are feeling. Even with such an initial state of total unity and transcendence, it is often helpful to go on to contemplate the questions, and perhaps record one's answers or comments, for post-session review.

Just as affirmations, or statements of intention, can be used as a bridge from one's ordinary state of consciousness to these heightened states, so can intentional affirmations be made during the empathogenic state that will apply to the subsequently re-established ordinary state. Individuals have made statements of intention in regard to questions of emotional attitude, of communication in relationships, of creative expression; even changes in diet, exercise, or life-style have been arrived at, decided, and later applied. During the state of heightened though balanced, emotional awareness, one can think clearly about the various options available, without the usual distortions caused by our emotional attractions or aversions. One can think about and feel the emotional implications of different courses of action. One can assess the probable emotional impact of things one might choose to say to a partner or friend, and one can modify one's expression so as to minimize the activation of the other's defensive or hostile reactions. One can hear things without getting hurt or angry, and one can say things without getting fearful or timid.

If the statements above sound "too good to be true," we can only respond that they are based on repeated experiences and observations of many hundreds of intelligent, articulate individuals. What usually strikes one is the profound simplicity of the empathogenic MDMA state. People often express this in the form of apparently banal statements, such as that one only needs love and all else falls into place, or that coming from the heart center, or from the Source, makes all other choices easy and right. What these observations and experiences imply is that with MDMA we have a substance with perhaps its greatest value and potential in the training of psychotherapists. Psychotherapists who have taken it frequently also report having insights into their clients' problems, as well as their own.

All of the various practices of meditation, of yoga, of guided imagery, of psychosynthesis, of shamanic journey work and of rebirthing breathing, can be performed while in this state. Most people who have attempted this have found it most effective to practice these methods either with low dosages of MDMA (50–100 mg), or toward the latter half of the session (after two or three hours). It is reported by many that such methods, which are essentially self-initiated and self-guided explorations of consciousness, are facilitated and amplified while in these states. People have reported that in the empathogenic state they experienced and understood for the first time, what the nature and efficacy of a given technique really was. Various forms of body-work, including massage, can also be amplified in their range and depth if the recipient's awareness has been sensitized by empathogens (again in lower dosages).

Process and Ritual for Group Sessions

Among the therapists and group leaders from whom the reports in this book have been collected, there appears to have evolved two basic types of approaches to group work. (We are speaking of group work whose focus and intention is serious self-exploration in a group context; ecstasy parties or "raves" are not being considered here). In one type of group, the participants have no interaction with one another during the session, although before and afterwards there is significant sharing of intentions and experiences. Each individual explores his or her own "trip," listening to music with earphones, and communicating if necessary only with the guides. In the other type of group, there is communication during the session, but in a scrupulously adhered to ritual fashion.

Some groups have experimented with night-time sessions, following the example of Central and South American shamanic cultures that use mushrooms or ayahuasca. However, since the onset of normal fatigue can appreciably shorten a session begun in the evening, others have preferred daytime sessions. Typically, a group will assemble on a Friday evening, talk and share their intentions with one another, and sleep that night in the same building. Starting the session in the morning, they continue until evening, sleep another night; and then do the final sharing, breaking of the fast, and celebration on the following morning (Sunday).

The particular substances used may also vary from group to group. In some, different participants may take different substances, including LSD, mushrooms, MDMA, or ketamine. In others, only MDMA may be used; or MDMA, followed three to four hours later by 2CB, in order to prolong the empathogenic state. Most therapists and group leaders agree that it is not wise to encourage someone to participate in a group experience who has not had previous individual experiences with the particular substance involved. The first time with any substance, including MDMA, may lead an individual to an intense verbal or physical expression of their feeling states. I have been with clients who, on their first experience with MDMA, literally could not stop talking. Another person spent a couple of hours repeatedly slapping his body on the chest, arms and back. This kind of behavior, which can be extremely distracting to others, can be difficult to stop on one's first exposure to a particular substance. In subsequent sessions one normally has much more choice in regard to expression. (These kinds of behavior could also be a function of an excessive dose for that particular individual).

In the kinds of groups in which talking is permitted, one common ritual practice is to use a talking-staff. This is adapted from the practices of the peyote sessions of the Native American Church, and is used in some non-drug healing circles, and in some political decision-making councils. One talks, or sings, only when one has the staff; then one speaks or sings from the heart and the other group members listen respectfully, without reaction, question or interpretation. The combination of intense inner experiences with the receptive attentiveness of the group, is a powerful, almost magnetic attracting force. This can draw someone's heart-felt expression through, in an often surprising manner. Sometimes group members choose, when they have the staff, not to talk, but simply to share a silent meditation. In these kinds of groups, a typical session might consist of 40 minutes of individual inner exploration, while listening to music, followed by a round of songs and sharings with the talking staff. In this way a rhythm develops in which internalized experience alternates with externalized expression.

An explicit agreement of strict confidentiality should always be made: anything that anyone either says, does or ingests, is agreed not to be discussed outside the circle of the group. This not only protects the individuals from unwanted gossip, or possible legal consequences, but also serves to build trust. As a result I have witnessed some truly extraordinary revelations being made in these groups. Similar agreements are used in other Native American groups, such as the sweat-lodge ceremony, so that each individual participating can feel completely confident that what he or she shares will not be shared outside the group. It is the group leader's responsibility to ensure that a level of trust exists in the group.

In such a group there is then no talking, or chatting separately among two or more members of the group. The integrity of the circle is maintained by participants either lying silently in a circle with their heads toward the center, or sitting on the same spot while the staff is being passed around. The energy that builds up in such a group is highly charged, and its power can be "used," as it were, by each individual to amplify his or her own intrapsychic process. It also can be used by the group to focus energy on planetary networks of light and consciousness as is done in many peace circles.

Besides the agreement on the structure of communication and confidentiality, agreements on touch and sexual behavior are also called for. Any sexual behavior in the group is discouraged; even in the case of couples who are in the group together; to engage in sexual behavior would be seen by the rest of the group as exclusive and as dissipating the energy. It should be understood, though, that sometimes the simple touch of a hand from one's neighbor can be the most profoundly re-assuring and comforting gesture.

Again, one needs to find a balance: inexperienced participants sometimes make the mistake of assuming that someone who is crying, sobbing, moaning or groaning, is somehow in need of help or comfort. A "comforter" may seek to make a painful experience go away (i.e., to placate) when the individual concerned is much more likely to want and cherish the opportunity to experience deeply-buried feelings for the first time. Just a simple touch, indicating presence and support if needed, is probably the most effective therapeutic aid in such situations.

Other kinds of rituals that have been adapted by some groups from shamanic tribal cultures include: at the beginning and end of the session finding a "power spot" outside, in silence, and meditating there before and after the session; or placing a blanket with ritual power objects that people have brought in the center, and letting these objects be "charged" during the session; offering prayers to the four directions, and the four elements (or rather the spirit or intelligence of those elemental powers). Group rebirthing, breathing work, or movement patterns such as Tai Chi have also been incorporated into some group rituals. Those kinds of group ritual activities usually work best in low-dosage sessions.

Follow-up and After-effects

An interesting question for many people concerns the extent to which the insights and changes of such experiences with empathogens are permanent. Is it possible to transfer the learning, the new attitudes and feelings, into one's everyday reality? Or, to put this question another way, what kind of behavior or personality changes occur in people after the deep states of consciousness of the kind described in this book?

From reviewing the work of therapists and guides who have witnessed sessions with MDMA and other empathogens, one is lead to the conclusion that there are two main kinds of outcomes. In one group of people there is no discernible outward change in behavior. The significant changes occurred in attitude, in emotional response to situations. They may discover that what they were doing was in line with their true spiritual purpose. They feel confirmed in their commitment; they have more compassion and true understanding. The second group are those who do see things in their life that they want to and can change, and they then proceed in a more or less systematic manner to bring about those changes. Some patterns that people have changed have ranged from physical symptoms, dietary habits, work habits and attitudes, to basic changes in world view, in religious or spiritual practice, or in fundamental career changes.

We have known some individuals that have had only one experience with MDMA, and have made major life-changes as a result of this one experience. Others find they may "need" three or four or five sessions, to clear out some basic problems. After that, they may find that the experience doesn't "take" any more; there is a kind of psychic tolerance. Alternatively, some feel that the space of the MDMA experience can be entered at will, without the substance, and do not have the major reorganizing that they experienced the first time.

The intention or set of the individual in taking the substance is also crucial with regard to the after-effects. The intention before the session affects experiences during it, and the intentions acknowledged and affirmed during the experience affect the long-term outcomes. Intention seems to function as a kind of bridge between states of consciousness.

It is also the impression of many therapists and observers that the empathogens, more than other psychedelics or hallucinogens, leave one with the ability to consciously recall the state of consciousness—to do a kind of voluntary, purposive "flashback." One therapist, for example, reported that clients could be asked to remember how they felt during their MDMA session, and then use that feeling of compassion and well-being to look at and deal with a troublesome issue in their current life. Some have used physical "anchoring" techniques, such as listening to the music they hear during their session, to bring them back into a momentary reliving of their experience. It's almost as if the doorway of the heart-center, once opened, stays open, or can be opened very easily again, by choice.

There is a feeling of being empowered to make conscious choices about the direction of one's life, and one's relationships, or work, or creativity, and that one can empathetically sense what the emotional consequences of one's choices will be. One can choose where one directs one's attention and focus of awareness. One woman reported feeling that there were paths that went out from the heart-center, and that she could choose which one was most appropriate for her; and not just take the one always taken, the traditional, expected path. Many possibilities open for those who have found themselves in this great gateway to the inner realms of light and beauty.

References for the Guidelines

Holland, Julie (Editor). (2001). *Ecstasy: The Complete Guide: A Comprehensive Look at the Risks and Benefits of MDMA.* South Paris, ME: Park Street Press.

Naranjo, C. (1975). *The Healing Journey-New Approaches to Consciousness.* New York, NY: Ballantine Books.

Shulgin, Alexander & Shulgin, Ann. (1991). *Pihkal: A Chemical Love Story.* Berkeley, CA: Transform Press.

Stolaroff, M. (2005). *The Secret Chief Revealed.* Santa Cruz, CA: MAPS.

Books & CDs by Ralph Metzner

Available from *Green Earth Foundation*

www.greenearthfound.org

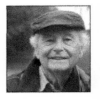

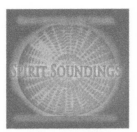

Spirit Soundings – *Music & Spoken Word CD*
Poems by **Ralph Metzner**
Music by **Kit Walker,** with **Michael Bransom, Doc Collins, Mariana Ingold**
2012. $20

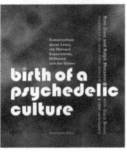

Birth of a Psychedelic Culture – *Conversations about Leary, the Harvard Experiments, Millbrook and the Sixties*
Ram Dass and **Ralph Metzner,** with **Gary Bravo**
Foreword by **John Perry Barlow**
Illustrated with numerous photographs. Commentaries by 15 other contributors.
Synergetic Press, Santa Fe, NM, 2010. 240 pp. $25.

Eye of the Seeress - Voice of the Poet
Visions – Poems – Prayers. In German and English. Selected and Translated by Ralph Metzner 2011, 88 pp. $20.

Sacred Mushroom of Visions – *Teonanácatl.* Scientific chapters and personal experience accounts. ed. by Ralph Metzner. Illustrated. Park Street Press, 2005. 294 pp. $20.

Sacred Vine of Visions – *Ayahuasca.* Scientific chapters and personal experience accounts. ed. by Ralph Metzner. Illustrated. Park Street Press, 2006. 264 pp. $20.

Green Psychology – *Transforming Our Relationship to the Earth.* With Foreword by Theodore Roszak and Epilogue by John Seed. Park Street Press, 1999. 229 pp. $20.

The Unfolding Self – *Varieties of Transformative Experience.* Twelve classic metaphors of psychospiritual transformation. Pioneer Imprints, 2010. 300 pp. $23.

The Well of Remembrance – *Rediscovering the Earth Wisdom Myths of Northern Europe.* With Foreword by Marija Gimbutas. Shambhala, 1994. 334 pp, $30.

Invocations. *Poetic invocations of nature spirits and spirit allies.* 16 pp booklet. $10.

Bardo Blues *and Other Songs of Liberation. (CD)* Original songs and prayers, composed and performed by Ralph Metzner. Produced and recorded by Kit Walker, additional vocals by Ella Zarum. $10

Books from the Series
THE ECOLOGY OF CONSCIOUSNESS
www.greenearthfound.org

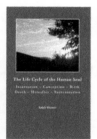

The Life Cycle of the Human Soul – *Incarnation - Conception - Birth - Death - Hereafter - Reincarnation*. In this book I discuss the experience of birth and of prenatal life, the soul's choosing of a human incarnation and the connection with familial ancestors. I also discuss the experience of death of the physical body and the soul's life in the intermediate realms before choosing rebirth into another life. 2011, 134 pp, $25.

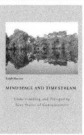

Mindspace and Timestream – *Understanding and Navigating Your States of Consciousness*. Each state of consciousness from the familiar to expansive spiritual states has its own distinctly different mindspace and time-stream. We need to learn how to use the positive states for spiritual growth and creative expression and navigate out of the contractive, unhealthy states of fear and rage, addictions and compulsions. 2009, 146 pp, $25.

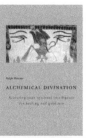

Alchemical Divination – *Accessing Your Spiritual Intelligence for Healing and Guidance*. Alchemy involves teachings and practices of physical, psychic and spiritual transformation. Divination is the practice of seeking healing and spiritual guidance from inner sources of wisdom and knowledge. The alchemical divination processes can help individuals obtain problem resolution and visionary inspiration for their life. 2009, 137 pp, $25.

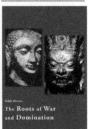

The Roots of War and Domination. I track these in the consequences of child abuse; in historical patterns of resource competition; and in mammalian predator behavior. I explore Buddhist, Atlantean, Nordic and Sumerian myths related to power and domination, and the complex and profound teachings of G.I. Gurdjieff. It is my hope that these explorations may lead to possibly healing solutions. 2008, 85 pp, $20.

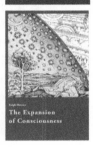

The Expansion of Consciousness. In part I, I describe how the teachings of alchemy were revived by C.G. Jung, who identified alchemical symbolism as the language of the psyche; and Albert Hofmann, who uncovered the secret link between Spirit and Matter. In part II, I describe how the counter-culture movements of the 1960s articulated an expansion of collective consciousness and a vision of society centered around humane and spiritual values. 2008, 83 pp, $20.

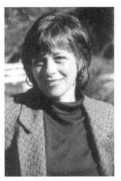